S0-DTB-295

Prentice-Hall Series in the Philosophy of Medicine

Samuel Gorovitz,
Series Editor

MAN, MIND, AND MORALITY: the ethics of behavior control, *Ruth Macklin*

ETHICAL ISSUES IN SUICIDE, *Margaret Pabst Battin*

NURSING PRACTICE: the ethical issues, *Andrew Jameton*

REPRODUCTIVE ETHICS, *Michael D. Bayles*

Reproductive

Prentice-Hall, Inc., Englewood Cliffs, New Jersey 07632

Ethics

MICHAEL D. BAYLES

Westminster Institute for Ethics and Human Values
London, Canada

Library of Congress Cataloging in Publication Data

BAYLES, MICHAEL D.
Reproductive ethics.

(Prentice-Hall series in the philosophy of medicine)
Includes bibliographies and index.
1. Human reproduction—Moral and ethical aspects.
I. Title. II. Series.
QP251.B34 1984   174'.2   83-17752
ISBN 0-13-773904-4

© 1984 by Prentice-Hall, Inc., Englewood Cliffs, New Jersey 07632

Printed in the United States of America

10 9 8 7 6 5 4 3 2 1

ISBN 0-13-773904-4

PRENTICE-HALL INTERNATIONAL, INC., *London*
PRENTICE-HALL OF AUSTRALIA PTY. LIMITED, *Sydney*
EDITORA PRENTICE-HALL DO BRASIL, LTDA., *Rio de Janeiro*
PRENTICE-HALL CANADA INC., *Toronto*
PRENTICE-HALL OF INDIA PRIVATE LIMITED, *New Delhi*
PRENTICE-HALL OF JAPAN, INC., *Tokyo*
PRENTICE-HALL OF SOUTHEAST ASIA PTE. LTD., *Singapore*
WHITEHALL BOOKS LIMITED, *Wellington, New Zealand*

To Teressa, Tony, Cynthia, and Krista

Contents

Cases and Scenarios

Preface
to the Series

It is a commonplace observation that there have been dramatic in-creases both in public and professional concern with questions of bioethics and in the role of philosophers in addressing those questions. Medical ethics is a well-established area of inquiry; not only does it include journals, wide-spread courses, professional specialists, and the other features of established fields, but philosophers now participate regularly in the deliberations of public agencies at both state and federal levels. Nonetheless, there is consid-erably more to the philosophy of medicine than medical ethics, and even within the area of medical ethics, there are many issues that have not been adequately explored.

The Prentice-Hall Series in the Philosophy of Medicine has been estab-lished in large measure in response to these two points. Some volumes in the series will explore philosophical aspects of medicine that are not primarily questions of ethics. They thereby contribute both to the subject matter of the philosophy of medicine and to an expanding appreciation of the breadth and diversity of the philosophy of medicine. Other volumes in the series will illuminate areas of ethical concern which, despite the recent prominence of medical ethics, have been inadequately considered.

Each volume is written by a philosopher, although none is written primarily for philosophers. Rather, the volumes are designed to bring the issues before an intelligent general readership, and they therefore presup-pose no specific background in either the philosophical literature or the literature of the specific areas of medical practice or health policy on which they focus.

The problems considered in this series are of widespread public impor-tance. We suffer from no delusions that philosophers hold the solutions; we do, however, share the conviction that these problems cannot be adequately addressed without an informed appreciation of their philosophical dimensions. We must always reach beyond philosophy in addressing problems in the world, but we should be wary of reaching without it. The volumes in this series are thus addressed to all those concerned with the practices and policies relating to medicine and health, and committed to considering such policies in a reflective and rational way.

SAMUEL GOROVITZ

Preface

This book represents the summary of my thinking and working on these issues since 1974. During that time, I received so many valuable insights from others that probably nothing of value is mine alone. However, it is possible to acknowledge only some of the debts that I have. A prime stimulus was a series of seminars during 1977 and 1978 in Montana on Ethical-Moral Dilemmas in the Medical Management of Genetic and Birth Defects and Mental Retardation. I wish to thank the organizer of the seminars, Philip Pallister, M.D., and the participants for enjoyable and educational experiences.

The only actual cases in this book are Cases 1.3, 1.5, 4.2, and 4.3. While some of the other cases were inspired by personal experiences or actual cases of others, especially cases presented at the Montana seminars, I have freely modified them to suit my purposes. The rest are simply fictional examples of common situations. I have tried to make all the cases as realistic as possible; the "scenarios," on the other hand, are pure invention.

Many persons directly assisted me in writing this book. A number of outstanding scholars gave freely of their time to read and critique an early draft. They are Bernard Dickens, John C. Fletcher, Barry Hoffmaster, Bruce Miller, and David B. Shurtleff. In each case, I have also greatly profited over the years from their writings and conversations. In addition, Samuel Gorovitz went beyond the call of duty of a series editor by twice throroughly reading and critiquing the manuscript for both content and style, and working especially hard to get the book into publication as quickly as possible. One could not ask for a better editor.

Deborah Rosen, my research assistant, spent many long hours trudging back and forth through snow and rain to the library to find materials. Laurie Bildfell, Nancy Margolis, and Hilda Tauber gave much needed editorial assistance, trying to make the text clear and to remove all my split infinitives. Janet Baldock and Ann Higgs efficiently and accurately typed several drafts of the complete manuscript.

Finally, the Social Sciences and Humanities Research Council of Canada, under grant no. 410-81-0717, provided the funds for the research and to release me from some teaching duties in order to complete the book. And the Westminster Institute for Ethics and Human Values provided the facilities and atmosphere conducive to the work.

M.D.B.

Introduction

Throughout most of history, human reproduction has been a natural process that people could not control. Many of the moral principles related to sex and human reproduction were based on the assumption of natural reproductive conditions. The changes brought by medical science have altered this assumption. Thus, it is necessary to rethink our views about the morality of human reproduction. New possibilities exist and moral principles must develop to deal with them.

For many complex reasons, most people in developed countries and many people in less developed ones are now having fewer children than did their ancestors a century ago. If people are going to have only one or two children, they are more concerned than ever that those children be healthy and normal. Moreover, people with conditions which would have prevented them from having children in the past now reasonably hope that they may be able to do so. In short, people typically hope to have a few normal, healthy genetic offspring.

During the last century, advances in medical science have significantly increased the chances that people will be able to do this. The last quarter century has seen the development of contraceptive techniques such as better surgical sterilization, contraceptive pills and injections, intra-uterine devices, and improved methods for determining the time of ovulation for the practice of periodic abstinence. New methods of conception have also been developed, such as artificial insemination and *in vitro* fertilization with embryo transfer ("test tube babies"). Methods are currently being sought to enable couples to choose the sex of their children. There are already a variety of techniques for determining whether a couple is likely to conceive a child with a genetic defect, or whether a fetus has a defect. Among these techniques are blood tests, fetoscopy (direct viewing of the fetus), ultrasound picturing, and amniocentesis (drawing fluid from the womb and testing it). Safer and more sophisticated abortion procedures have been developed.

Childbirth itself has undergone many medical changes. A century ago most births were at home; most are now hospital births, supervised by physicians who often use new technologies to monitor fetal heart beat and stress. Finally, new medical procedures help cure or alleviate defects in newborn infants. Many highly premature infants who would have died decades ago now survive and thrive.

The new possibilities in human reproduction have raised the hopes and fears of many people. While many people now hope to have fewer children, others fear the widespread violation of traditional moral principles, the harmful side effects of contraceptive pills and other contraceptive techniques, or the compulsory sterilization of large numbers of people deemed unfit to reproduce. Infertile couples can now hope to have a child of their own, but others fear the consequences of the new methods of reproduction for the family, children, and society. Many people hope that they will be able to determine their child's sex and have the boy or girl they have always wanted, while others fear that renewed sexism and an alteration of society will result. Many people now hope that they can avoid having a child with a serious genetic defect, while others fear that society will use genetic screening to deprive people of the chance of having children or to try to create a race of "perfect people." Many women now demand control of their bodies to avoid unwanted pregnancies, but other people perceive abortion as the killing of living babies. While many people believe that medical advances have made childbirth safer and easier, others fear that modern obstetrical techniques have deprived women (and men) of rewarding personal experiences and psychological bonding with their children, and have increased male dominance over female reproduction. Many parents have been given hope that premature or ill newborns can survive, but some people fear that the lives of severely damaged newborns are miserable and unnecessarily prolonged. Finally, many people hope, and others fear, that the future will bring new methods of reproduction in which genetic traits can be ordered at will, people can have offspring genetically identical with themselves, crosses between human beings and other species can be produced, defects can be cured before birth, and gestation can occur outside of human bodies.

Personal, Ethical, and Policy Standards

In this context of hope and fear, moral issues must be carefully examined. One important consideration is the distinction between personal ideals and ethics. Everyone has personal values or ideals that guide his or her conduct. I, for example, have an ideal of a good philosopher which I strive to attain; but I do not expect everyone to have that ideal. Ethical principles and standards are a different matter; I do expect people to conform to them. Ethical beliefs and standards are used to evaluate the conduct both of oneself and of others. It does not make sense to say, "I believe abortion is wrongful killing of innocent human beings, but it makes no difference to me whether or not people do it." We think other people should conform to ethical standards, and although it does not follow that we should or do impose them on others, we do judge that others are better or worse, depending upon whether they conform to the standards we hold. We praise or blame them for adhering to or violating those standards, although we may not always express it.

While ethical standards are used to evaluate the conduct of others, they are not necessarily imposed on others by coercion or by law. Policy standards are different in that they involve the use of the state or other organizations to get people to conform. A large variety of government techniques can be used to get people to act in desired ways—punishment, administrative regulation, allowing suits for damages, taxation, and paying people. Other policies are supported by other organizations, such as hospitals and professional associations. So while policy standards are also used to evaluate the conduct of others, they go beyond ethical standards by involving the use of power to obtain conformity.

Of course, policy standards do not necessarily rest on ethical ones. For example, in Canada the law requires that all food be sold by metric weights and measures, but in the United States pounds and ounces are used and the metric system is optional. Although legal control is needed to maintain common standards, the choice between the English and the metric systems rests on economic and other considerations, not ethical ones.

The differences between personal, ethical, and policy standards can readily be seen with respect to sterilization. Some people find the idea of being sterilized personally abhorrent and would never voluntarily undergo it; however, they do not regard sterilization as unethical or think it should be illegal. Other people regard sterilization for contraceptive purposes as ethically wrong (and therefore would not undergo it themselves), but do not think it should be illegal. And a few people believe that sterilization should be officially controlled, that, for example, its use in hospitals should be restricted to medical indications, such as removal of diseased material.

Moral Questions and Arguments

Moral analysis aims to bring about agreement by the use of rational argument. Rational discussion and argument are not guaranteed to bring about agreement—people are not always rational and there might not even be a rational solution. Nonetheless, most people try to have rational beliefs, but a recurrent problem has been precisely how and to what extent reason can be brought to bear on moral problems.

To be rational is to use logic and information as the basis for one's beliefs and attitudes. The fundamental requirement of logic is consistency, and rational people do not believe logically inconsistent claims, for example, that capital punishment is justifiable but that it is always wrong to kill another member of the human species. Besides deductive reasoning, based on consistency, rationality also uses inductive logic or scientific reasoning.

All relevant available information must be used in making a rational decision. Information is relevant if, by the use of logical reasoning, the information can affect the strength of reasons for deciding one way rather than another. In the broadest sense, information is available if and only if it is publicly ascertainable, that is, people can get the information. But of course, for a variety of reasons, one cannot always have all publicly ascertainable information. A decision may have to be made before the information can be obtained, or the costs of getting it may be prohibitive. Nonetheless, the goal is to obtain all the relevant information one can. Finally, one can only use available information, and the information available may not be correct. For example, present information indicates that children born by *in vitro* fertilization are little more likely than children conceived naturally to have genetic defects. However, further scientific study might prove that wrong. All one can do is use the currently available information and allow for the possibility that it might be incorrect.

To determine whether one's desires, personal standards, and ethical and policy values are rational, one asks whether one would hold them if all the relevant available information and logic were brought to bear on them.[1] Some things are desired or valued instrumentally—that is, because they are believed to lead to other valued things. If instrumentally desired things are not likely to bring about the valued state, desiring them is not rational. Other things are desired or valued for their own sake; they are considered to be intrinsically valuable and we can call desires for them intrinsic desires. Sometimes such desires are not rational because they are incompatible with other, stronger desires, or because they rest on beliefs about the desired object that are contrary to the best available information. Also, people are sometimes mistaken about what they value for its own sake. For example, many people discover that although they thought they loved someone, instead they merely wanted companionship or perhaps they wanted to have someone do things for them. To avoid such mistakes, in rationally determining whether things are intrinsically valuable, one must consider only those factors which are necessarily involved. Finally, sometimes good reasons can be given for not personally desiring something; it would contribute little or nothing to one's life, for example.

In considering personal values, one is primarily concerned with what their realization would mean for one's own life. Different rational people can have different personal values. When considering ethical and policy values, one must consider what it would be like for them to be realized in society. The social dimension is necessary because these are standards for evaluating others as well as oneself.

Besides values (and disvalues), morality also includes norms of conduct, that is, guidelines about how people should or should not act. The general question is whether a person with all relevant available information and only rational desires, who used logic, would accept these norms for a society in which that person was to live. To accept a norm is to be willing to use it to evaluate one's own conduct as well as that of others, and to be interested in seeing it adopted or accepted by most others in society. The society in question is the largest for which that norm or principle would be accepted.

Various types of considerations can be involved in bringing the relevant available information to bear on these questions. One type is what the consequences would be of most people acting in some manner, for example,

---

[1]The view briefly described here is basically that in Richard B. Brandt, *A Theory of The Good and The Right* (Oxford: Clarendon Press, 1979).

determining the sex of their children at conception. Another type of consideration is how the norm conforms with other norms one would accept. Some norms follow from more general ones together with certain facts. When that is not so, a norm can be justified by showing that it helps realize basic ethical or policy values such as privacy.

Because of the differences between ethical and policy norms, justifications of one are not necessarily justifications of the other. Ethical norms are supported by the praise and blame of others, and by being taught so that the members of society are motivated to conform to them, and to feel shame or guilt if they do not. Policy norms are used to control conduct by governmental or organizational power to prevent their violation and enforce conformity. Consequently, one may be willing to let others criticize one's conduct if they think it incorrect, but not be willing to let the government regulate it. For example, I may be willing to allow my relatives to complain and think poorly of me for not having more offspring, but not be willing to have the government force me to have children. Indeed, decisions regarding reproduction are generally considered to be just this type of conduct: appropriately evaluated by ethics but not by law.

Aims and Method

In the rest of this book, we shall examine the moral issues raised by people desiring to have only a few healthy, genetically normal offspring and the medical advances affecting their chances of doing so. We shall not examine the broad related issues of global population, since that has been done elsewhere.[2] The book attempts to illustrate how moral analysis can clarify issues, assess arguments and reasons for various positions, indicate well-supported values and norms relevant to decisions, and sometimes provide intellectual or institutional procedures for decision making. We will keep personal, ethical, and policy standards distinct.

To determine whether desires or values are rational, we shall consider whether one would hold them if all relevant information and logic were brought to bear on them. We shall consider intrinsic desires (wanting things for their own sake) irrational if (1) they rest on mistakes about relevant available information, especially the character of what is desired; (2) they rest on failure to distinguish one object of desire from another which is primarily desired; (3) the fulfillment of personal desires would not contribute anything to one's life experience; or (4) other good reasons can be given for not having them, for example, that acting on them would prevent fulfillment of other, stronger rational desires. Instrumental desires are irrational if their fulfillment will not significantly contribute to the fulfillment of intrinsic desires.

To determine whether norms are correct, we ask whether, if one had no irrational desires, had all relevant information, and used logic, one would accept them for a society in which one was to live. Acceptable norms must be supported by sound arguments showing that they contribute to the real-

[2]See Michael D. Bayles, *Morality and Population Policy* (University, Ala.: University of Alabama Press, 1980).

ization of ethical or policy values. Sound arguments are those that are logically valid, with premises that, on the basis of available information, are probably true. Norms are unacceptable if (1) the arguments for them are not sound; (2) they are logically inconsistent with other more important norms; or (3) they would prevent the realization of values more basic than those they would promote.

Throughout, the underlying question concerns what rational persons would accept as values or norms. The arguments and conclusions are addressed to readers as rational persons.

There are basically three types of questions to be asked about various aspects of human reproduction: (1) What desires and values are rational? (2) Given rational desires and values, what ethical norms can be accepted? (3) Given rational desires and values, what policy norms are acceptable? These three questions need to be asked about almost all of the methods and technologies mentioned above—contraception, conception, sex preselection, genetic screening, abortion, methods of childbirth, treatment of defective newborns, and possible future methods of human reproduction and fetal treatment.

One substantive moral assumption is implicit in our method: Freedom is a basic value of rational persons.[3] This is partly implied by the assumption that ethical and policy norms will not be accepted by rational persons unless good reasons are offered for them. However, the assumption is stronger. The presumption is always in favor of freedom; those who want to limit it by ethical or policy norms must carry the burden of persuasion. To support an ethical or policy norm limiting conduct, sound arguments must be offered to show that the value of freedom is outweighed.

[3]For a defense of this assumption, see *ibid.*, pp. 26–27; and Michael D. Bayles, *Principles of Legislation: The Uses of Political Authority* (Detroit: Wayne State University Press, 1978), pp. 71–83.

CHAPTER 1

Contraception
and Conception

Contraception

Case 1.1 Alice and Bob have been married for ten years and have two children, ages nine and four. Bob is thirty-one years old and Alice is twenty-eight. They have more or less decided that they do not want any more children—at least Bob is sure he does not want any more, although Alice is not so definite about it. Both of Alice's pregnancies were difficult, and she was advised not to have more children. Alice and Bob have used contraceptive methods, primarily the pill, both to space the births of their children and to limit the number of children they have. The prospect of Alice's taking contraceptive pills until menopause is not attractive due to the risks of side effects, which increase with age and length of use. Consequently, Bob is considering a sterilization.

This case is not unusual, and few people think that it raises any ethical problems. Most people believe that contraception is ethically permissible, and most North Americans practice it. Nonetheless, this case raises basic ethical issues that are fundamental to many reproductive questions. A general question of reproductive ethics is whether people have a duty to reproduce. Even if they do not, is reproduction a good thing, or is it morally neutral? Another issue concerns methods of contraception; some people believe that some forms of contraception are ethically wrong.

A Duty to Reproduce

Probably the most pervasive argument for a duty to reproduce stems from natural law theory, which bases ethical principles on empirical features of the world. People should do good and avoid evil,[1] but what is good or evil? The central premise of natural law ethics is that good and evil can be determined by the purposes inherent in people's natural inclinations. These purposes establish ends, or *goods,* for humans that conduct ought to respect. For example, humans, along with other animals and even inanimate things, act to continue or preserve their existence. From this, it follows that life is a fundamental good or value.

The central natural law argument about reproduction can be set out as follows:

1. Good ought to be pursued and evil avoided.
2. Good ends are those towards which people are naturally inclined.
3. People are naturally inclined to sexual intercourse.
4. A natural purpose of sexual intercourse is reproduction.
5. Therefore, reproduction ought to be pursued in sexual acts.
6. To act intentionally against the good of reproduction is evil and ought to be avoided.

The last two steps in this argument are very important for ethical issues of human reproduction. Step 5 establishes what is often called a "duty to procreate," and step 6 is the basis for judging some forms of contraception wrong.

The duty to reproduce expressed in step 5 is not one that every individual must act to fulfill. The object of reproduction is continuation of the species, and not everyone must have children to fulfill this end.[2] If enough people have children to continue the species, others can ethically remain celibate. However, because reproduction is a good, and intentionally to frustrate a natural end of an act is wrong, it is wrong intentionally to prevent the natural outcome of intercourse by using contraceptive devices.

Several objections can be made to this argument. One problem is how one determines the ends of natural inclinations. For example, why must reproduction be an end of sexual intercourse? Natural law theorists reply that the natural ends of an activity or inclination are those things which it alone can accomplish or can accomplish better than anything else. Even though most instances of intercourse do not result in pregnancy, still, in nature that is the only way human beings can reproduce. Even if this response is plausible here, in many other cases it is not clear that there is an end which can be produced only by acting on a specific inclination.

A more basic objection criticizes step 2 in the argument. Why, it may be asked, are those ends towards which people are naturally inclined good? Some psychologists have held that people are naturally inclined to aggression or death. If that were true, we would surely not conclude that harming and injuring others is good! Natural law theory assumes that if people are naturally inclined to act in some way, then that must produce some good. If the universe was made by God and He would not endow creatures with bad inclinations, then one would have reason to accept the assumption. However, considering that the evolutionary process excludes only traits and inclinations inconsistent with survival through the age of reproduction, there is

[1]St. Thomas Aquinas, *Summa Theologica,* 1–11, q. 94, a. 2.

[2]Aquinas, *Summa Theologica,* 11–11, q. 152, a. 2 and ad. 1.

no reason to assume that people's natural inclinations are all for good ends. Consequently, with present information, no reason exists to accept the principle that the ends of natural inclinations are good. Thus natural law theory does not provide an acceptable basis for morality.

Nonetheless, there may be other reasons for believing it good for people to reproduce. If people's lives contain intrinsic good, then it is good that people live. At this point, it does not matter what one takes to be intrinsically good in people's lives—pleasure, happiness, knowledge, or capacities for communication and love. So long as this good is found in the lives of people (and is not outweighed by bad), then their existence is good. If such a life is called a valuable life, then a valuable life is a good thing. Bringing about a valuable life by reproducing is then a good thing to do, provided greater harm is not also produced.

Another moral theory, utilitarianism, might at this point appear to support a duty to procreate. The *act utilitarian* version holds that an act is permissible if and only if it produces at least as much net intrinsic good as any alternative act one could perform. If an act produces more net good than any alternative, one has a duty to perform it. Net intrinsic good is simply intrinsic good less intrinsic bad. If anything one can do (including doing nothing) produces more bad than good, then one ought to perform the act that produces the least net bad. This view would imply a duty to reproduce if reproducing would produce more good than not reproducing or any other alternative act.

There are sound reasons for not accepting act utilitarianism as a fundamental ethical principle for a society in which one expects to live.[3] First, people are quite likely to fail to perform such utilitarian acts, and this can result in guilt feelings. Second, it is often quite difficult to determine which act will produce the most good; others are also likely to be mistaken about when people could so act, and falsely blame them for not producing good. Third, it is difficult to determine what other people will do so as to plan one's own conduct in reliance on that. A fourth and very important reason is that people would have little opportunity to simply do the things they want to do. Most, if not all of the time, they would have to worry about whether they should be doing another act that would produce more net good. All of these sound reasons can be advanced for not accepting as an ethical principle one that requires people always to do the most net good.

Nor should one accept a principle requiring one to reproduce, even though it might produce much good and would not occupy all of one's time. A number of reasons (which also show that even act utilitarianism would not always require one to have children) can be given against this principle. Many people do not want to have children, and the duty to reproduce would impose much unhappiness upon them. If from a sense of duty they did have unwanted children, they probably would not be good parents. The children would be much less happy and their lives less likely to contain intrinsic good than if they had good parents. By refraining from having children, people do not cause them any suffering; because unconceived children do not exist, they cannot desire to exist. In the world today, more than enough children

[3]See Richard B. Brandt, *A Theory of The Good and The Right* (Oxford: Clarendon Press, 1979), pp. 271–77.

are being conceived to ensure that the species will continue; indeed, over-population may threaten the continuation of human beings, at least human beings who have valuable lives. Perhaps in some dire situation, for example, in the event of a nuclear war with a few survivors, there might be reasons to accept a duty to reproduce, but at present and for the foreseeable future there are not.

We have examined the two most common ethical arguments for a duty to reproduce. Neither of them is sound. As the burden of proof is on those who would impose duties and obligations, in the absence of a sound argument for such a duty, it must be rejected. In this case, we have seen that there are even good reasons against such a duty.

Contraceptive Methods

The discussion so far has established that Alice and Bob will not do anything wrong by not having more children. Indeed, they would not have done anything wrong had they not had any. This leaves the question of whether they acted wrongly in using the contraceptive methods they did, and whether it is ethically acceptable for Bob to be sterilized.

The natural law argument concludes that intentionally acting against the good of reproduction is wrong. While that argument was rejected, we determined that although there is no duty to reproduce, reproducing valuable lives is a good thing. This conclusion might be sufficient for the natural law argument against contraception. Sexual intercourse, it is claimed, has the purpose of reproduction, which must be pursued for intercourse to be ethically permissible. (It also has the purpose of expressing marital love.) If couples use artificial contraceptive methods, then they intentionally act contrary to the good of reproduction. The rhythm method of not having intercourse while the woman is fertile is, however, permissible. With it, a couple intentionally performs an act open to reproduction although they know that it will not occur.[4]

Two different questions can be asked about this argument. First, is it possible consistently to hold that use of contraceptive devices is wrong, but that use of the rhythm method is permissible? Second, is it wrong to use contraceptive devices? The argument for the difference between the rhythm and other methods depends on the distinction between intending an infertile act and intending a fertile act when one knows and desires that it will not result in pregnancy. This distinction is morally irrelevant. In both cases, couples have the same desire—not to have children—and know that pregnancy will not result. Neither act produces any harm or consequences that the other one does not. In one case a couple has intercourse in circumstances that prevent pregnancy, and in the other they arrange the circumstances to prevent pregnancy. Even if two different descriptions apply to the acts, the descriptions do not affect anything that is morally important, because it is not wrong to deny the reproductive purpose. Although reproducing valuable lives is a good thing, it does not support a duty to procreate

[4]See G. E. M. Anscombe, "Contraception and Chastity," in *Ethics and Population,* ed. Michael D. Bayles (Cambridge, Mass.: Schenkman Publishing Company, Inc., 1976), pp. 146–48.

which makes it wrong not to pursue that purpose. Without premise 5 in the natural law argument, conclusion 6 does not follow. Consequently, one does no wrong in intentionally performing an infertile act of sexual intercourse, that is, in using contraceptive devices. Alice and Bob have not acted wrongly by using the contraceptive methods they have.

The remaining question is whether sterilization would be different. One might argue that it constitutes making oneself permanently incapable of pursuing the good of reproduction. One might also consider it a form of self-mutilation. Nonetheless, if there is no duty to reproduce, then making oneself incapable of reproducing is not wrong. Nor is it a gross form of mutilation; it is merely depriving oneself of one capacity in order, perhaps, better to enjoy and perform others—to enjoy sexual intercourse without fear of pregnancy and to ensure that one does not have to deprive one's children of care by caring for another sibling.

The burdens of any ethical principle requiring or prohibiting methods of contraception would far outweigh the good that might result. Consequently, only personal considerations are left for Alice and Bob to use in deciding on contraceptive methods. Some methods are more reliable than others; some carry greater risks of side effects, such as perforation of the uterus by an intrauterine device or blood clots from use of contraceptive pills; some are less likely to be reversible than others—for example, sterilization. Individuals have different desires and preferences and are in many different situations; it is best to let them choose in light of their own concerns.

Artificial Insemination by Donor

Case 1.2 Carrie and Doug have been married for four years. They both want children and started trying to have them a year after they married. When after a year Carrie was not pregnant, they went to a doctor. After a number of tests, Doug was found to be sterile. This was a serious blow to both Carrie and Doug, but they still wanted to raise children. They went to an adoption agency and were told that if they were found to be acceptable parents it would be about six years before they could get a child. They filled out the application forms and a year later were approved for adoption. However, they are now both twenty-eight years old and do not want to wait another five years to adopt. After considerable thought and discussion, they return to the fertility clinic and both request that Carrie be artificially inseminated with the sperm of another male. This way they will not have to wait five years with no assurance of getting a child even then. Their child will at least be genetically related to Carrie, who will carry it to term.

After obtaining the consent of both Carrie and Doug, the physician at the clinic chooses a donor with the same general physical features as Doug—moderate height, blue eyes, and brown hair. He also takes a medical history of the donor and his family for indications of transmissible genetic defects and does a blood test for Rh compatibility. The donor (who remains anonymous to Carrie and Doug) produces fresh semen by masturbation, for which he is paid $50.00 by the clinic. A nurse injects the semen into Carrie's vagina. This occurs twice the first month, but Carrie does not become pregnant. At the end of the second month, she is pregnant.

Artificial insemination by donor, or AID, has been practiced for most of this century. In the United States, perhaps 10,000 children are conceived each year by this technique.[5] The case of Carrie and Doug is typical. AID is primarily used to overcome male sterility. Increasingly, this sterility is the result of voluntary sterilization in a previous marriage. Another reason, which is becoming more prominent, is to avoid the possibility of transmitting a genetic defect, either because the man and woman are both carriers of a recessive gene, or because the man has been exposed to radiation in a medical treatment or at work. A variation for men with low sperm counts (AIH, or artificial insemination by husband) is to collect several samples of semen from the man and pool the sperm in one insemination; but our focus is on the more common practice of using donor sperm. A few sperm banks exist that sell frozen donor sperm, but usually fresh semen, often from medical students, is used. Donors are usually screened and paid a modest fee for each ejaculate. AID is not always successful, and when it is, inseminations over several months may be necessary before a pregnancy occurs.

Desires to Have Children

To evaluate AID, we must first evaluate the rationality and importance of desires to have children. Let us begin by distinguishing between the desires to beget, bear, and rear children. The desire to beget, as used here, is wanting to have genetic offspring, that is, children stemming from one's sperm or ova. The desire to bear children is one that (at least at present) only women can reasonably have; it is the desire to gestate and deliver a fetus at term. The desire to rear children is wanting to have the parental role in raising them. Medical science has now made fulfillment of all the various combinations of these desires possible. Previously, people could adopt and rear children they did not beget or bear. Through new techniques discussed later in this chapter, women can now bear but not beget, or beget but not bear children. Not only have modern contraceptive methods separated sexual intercourse from reproduction, but reproduction has now been separated from sexual intercourse, and various parts of reproduction have been separated from each other.

One of Carrie and Doug's reasons for using AID is so that the child will be genetically related to one of them. As explained in the Introduction, a desire or value is irrational if a person with all available relevant information using logic and scientific reasoning would not have it. In considering whether an intrinsic desire (for something in itself) is rational, one must be careful to consider only the factual situation necessary to fulfill that desire, excluding all other conditions. Having genetic offspring does not necessarily involve bearing or rearing a child. It requires only that one's sperm or ovum

[5]Martin Curie-Cohen, Lesleigh Luttrell, and Sander Shapiro, "Current Practice of Artificial Insemination by Donor in the United States," *New England J. Med.*, 300, no. 11 (1979), 588.

contribute one-half the genetic makeup of an existing human being. The desire to beget could be fulfilled by merely donating sperm or ova successfully used in conception. No experience is necessarily involved beyond making the donation, and for women that would probably occur under anesthesia. Moreover, one must discount the satisfaction one would have from knowing that one's donation was used, because that satisfaction is dependent on one's having the desire. That is, one would not have the satisfaction unless one had the desire, so it cannot be a reason for having the desire.

The question, thus, is whether a person who reflected on these facts would have a desire to beget for its own sake; that is, whether begetting is intrinsically valuable. That many people do in fact desire to beget is not very relevant to answering this question, for few if any of them have isolated what is involved in the fulfillment of a desire to beget. People generally combine begetting and rearing, because they usually occur together. Also, as discussed below, their desires may be culturally conditioned. Personal desires for things for their own sake are for desirable experiences; consequently, as noted in the Introduction, they are irrational if their fulfillment will not contribute to one's life experiences. Begetting does not necessarily involve any experience, and if it does, the experience is minimal. It seems unlikely that one who fully grasped what is involved and reflected on it would have such a desire. If so, the desire to beget for its own sake is not rational.

Even if the desire to beget for its own sake is irrational, one might object, begetting might contribute to the value of bearing and rearing. That is, people might rationally prefer bearing or rearing a child that is genetically theirs to one that is not. However, one must ask what the genetic element will add. What is different in bearing or rearing one's genetic offspring from another child? The experiences themselves need not be any different, except for the thought that the child is or is not genetically one's own. Many people have raised children in the erroneous belief that the children were their genetic offspring when they were not, so the only difference seems to be the belief. Moreover, if the genetic relation were important, it would imply that adoptive parents cannot have as valuable experiences of child rearing as natural parents, which seems false. In short, due to cultural conditioning, most people think that rearing their genetic offspring is better than rearing children who are not genetically theirs, but any difference seems to stem solely from the belief.

Even if these arguments do not persuade one that a desire to beget for its own sake is irrational, the arguments in the rest of the book that use this premise need not be rejected. Those arguments primarily involve the claim that fulfillment of a desire to beget cannot override other concerns, such as risk of harm to offspring. Surely the preceding arguments show that even if rational, a desire to beget is not of major importance. Although I shall continue to use the stronger claim that a desire to beget is irrational, those who disagree can substitute the weaker claim that it is not of great importance.

The desire to beget can still be a rational, instrumental one; that is, it can be rational to desire to beget because it leads to the fulfillment of other desires. Indeed, the desire to beget is usually instrumentally rational, for it is normally the easiest way to obtain children to bear or rear. Historically, a number of reasons have supported an instrumental desire to have genetic offspring independent of bearing and rearing, but the reasons are unsound and do not support the claim that such a desire is instrumentally rational. One prominent reason was to have someone to inherit property. Traditionally, in Western Europe and North America, property passed to the first male heir; but today one can dispose of one's property by will to whomever one chooses. Another reason has been to continue the family name, but begetting does not guarantee that the name will be continued, and adopted children can also continue the name. Finally, some people believe that by begetting, a part of them continues, resulting in a sort of immortality. However, this is not continued conscious existence. Moreover, any offspring will derive half their genetic endowment from another person and be as much a continuation of that person as of oneself. Each individual is unique (even genetically identical twins have different personalities); no one is the incarnation of someone else. Besides, it takes an overblown ego to think that the continuation of one's self is a magnificent gift to society. Thus, while begetting can be instrumental to other goals, it is not necessary for them.

Next, consider the rationality of the desire to bear a child, that is, to carry a fetus and deliver at term. To fulfill that desire the fetus need not be one's genetic offspring, and in fact one need not ever see the child. Certainly the experience of bearing a child is longer and more varied than that of begetting a child. Many women do not find the experience of pregnancy intrinsically desirable, because of morning sickness, back strain, and so forth; yet some women do find the experience rewarding and enjoyable. Of course, the question is not whether a woman has the desire to bear, but whether with full information and reflection she would so desire. Some women who long to carry a child and give birth may be confusing the desire to bear for its own sake with a desire to bear as instrumental in having a child to rear; but this probably does not apply to all women. Thus, it is probable that some fully informed women would have an intrinsic desire to bear and that the desire is rational. Just as it is not irrational for some people to like cauliflower while others do not, so it is not irrational for some women to desire to bear a child while others do not.

Finally we consider the desire to rear a child. The experience of rearing a child is the longest and most complex of the three. It involves all the activities of nurturing a child from infancy to adulthood, including such disparate activities as feeding, diapering, playing with, teaching, punishing, and so on. A great deal of time, energy, money, and psychological stress can be involved. Nonetheless, there are many enjoyable aspects: for example, cuddling infants and watching them learn to crawl, walk, talk, and develop in other ways. Many people find these activities on the whole valuable. Surely a fully informed, reflective person could have an intrinsic desire to rear children. Moreover, since rearing a child is a longer and more challenging activity than bearing one, the desire to rear a child is probably stronger and more important to the person's life than the desire to bear one.

Both Carrie and Doug have rational desires to rear a child. Carrie's desire to bear a child is also rational. Doug's desire to beget a child is irrelevant, because it cannot be fulfilled in any case. While Carrie can and does beget, her desire to do so is probably not rational.

Ethical Analysis

Determining the rationality and relative importance of desires is a necessary preliminary to ethical analysis. According to the method used in this book, correct ethical principles are those that persons with rational desires and all relevant available information would accept for a society in which they expect to live. If a desire is irrational it would not motivate such people to accept an ethical principle; but it cannot be assumed that everyone in that society will have only rational desires. People would not necessarily be prohibited from acting on irrational desires, however; the burden of proof falls upon those who wish to restrict conduct ethically, and more is needed than to show that conduct stems from an irrational desire. Nonetheless, activity fulfilling rational desires would be evaluated as better than activity fulfilling irrational desires. Consequently, while not necessarily prohibiting the fulfillment of irrational desires, rational persons would not be likely to be much concerned to assist in fulfilling them.

Two general arguments might be offered against the ethical permissibility of AID. One argument is that because AID is an artificial method of conception rather than natural sexual intercourse, it is wrong just as "artificial" contraceptive methods are wrong. However, the natural law argument against contraceptive devices was shown to be unsound, and in any case, that argument cannot be applied to AID. The central premise of the argument against contraception is that it involves intentionally acting contrary to the good of reproduction; but AID acts in furtherance of, not contrary to, the good of reproduction.

The second argument is that AID wrongfully separates reproduction from a loving sexual act. Just as reproduction is one purpose of sexual intercourse, the expression of marital love is another. Every sexual act must express marital love and be open to reproduction.[6] Consequently, reproduction should not occur except in loving sexual acts.

This argument is unsound. Even if we accept the premise that acts of sexual intercourse must be open to reproduction, it does not follow that reproduction should occur only from sexual intercourse. Moreover, even if reproduction should occur only within a context of marital love, the point of that requirement is the nurturance of offspring. Such nurturance does not depend on the sexual act itself. The argument confuses the biological act with the familial context. At least in cases such as that of Carrie and Doug, the child will be nurtured in the context of a loving marriage. Extreme proponents of this argument contend that AID amounts to adultery—the uniting of sperm and ovum of two people one of whom is married but not to the other. Such a view transforms marriage into a concern with genetic material, rather than a loving relationship between persons. But the real harm in adultery lies in its destructive effects on this loving relationship.

The issue of adultery does relate to a more important and difficult issue, namely, the respective parental rights and duties of the woman's husband and of the semen donor. Donors usually contribute on an implicit or explicit condition that they will not have responsibilities toward any chil-

---

[6]See Pope Paul VI, "Humanae Vitae," in *Philosophy & Sex,* ed. Robert Baker and Frederick Elliston (Buffalo: Prometheus Books, 1975), p. 137.

dren produced and that the children will not have any claims against them—for financial support, for example. Indeed, were they liable to such parental duties, most men would probably refuse to be a donor.

No strong reason exists to prohibit determination of the rights and responsibilities of donors by an agreement made prior to donation. Usually, this means a donor has no duties to any offspring and is guaranteed anonymity, although the agreement could provide otherwise. An objection to this procedure is that children are deprived of the possibilities of inheriting from donors or knowing who their genetic fathers are. The question of inheritance and fathering need not be crucial in cases like that of Carrie and Doug. If Doug has the responsibilities of fatherhood and the child can claim them from him, then the child does have a father for nurturing and support; that is, the child is not deprived of a social father. Moreover, if the genetic father will donate only if he remains anonymous and has no duties, then these are the only conditions under which this child can exist; had someone else's sperm been used, *this* child would not have existed. (The matter of children knowing the identity of their genetic parents is considered below.)

Suppose, however, Carrie was artificially inseminated without Doug's consent. Should he then have parental responsibilities? If Carrie became pregnant by sexual intercourse with another man, the law would presume Doug to be the father unless he could prove he was not (which Doug could do). A fundamental ethical principle is involved here: No one should involuntarily have parental responsibilities, and people should have the opportunity to make a fully voluntary and informed choice to acquire them. The first half of this principle prohibits completely involuntary parenthood. The second half establishes the goal of providing people the opportunity to make fully voluntary and informed choices to become parents. It does not, however, imply that if people do not use the opportunity they are absolved of parental responsibility. Indeed, it is wrong to fail to make as voluntary and informed a choice as is possible, because the well-being of others (children) depends on it.

The reason for this principle of reproductive freedom is that parental responsibilities and rights are significant burdens and privileges which can greatly affect people's lives. People desire to have control over the major aspects of their lives, and there is no reason to think this desire is irrational. If people are to have control over their lives, then they should have control over the reproductive aspect. Consequently, this principle of reproductive freedom is a fundamental one for a society in which one expects to live; indeed, an ethical code that does not contain this principle is likely to be unacceptable. Hence, the consent of a woman's husband to AID is ethically required if he is to have parental responsibilities.

Carrie and Doug's reason for AID is the most common one, but an increasingly important reason for its use is to avoid passing on genetic defects. If both husband and wife are carriers of a recessive gene for some disease, such as sickle cell anemia which often results in a painful, early death, they have a 25 percent chance of transmitting the disease to their offspring. If this is the reason for using AID, it would be tragic if the donor was also a carrier of the recessive gene.

Ethically, how much should donors be screened for genetic defects?

The screening in Carrie and Doug's case is typical,[7] but one must ask whether it is sufficient. Clearly it is ethically wrong to donate semen or to use semen if one knows that a serious genetic defect is likely to be transmitted. It is prima facie wrong to take a substantial risk that an unborn child will have a significant defect. (This principle regarding risk to the unborn is justified in Chapter 2, where it is central.) Such a risk can always be avoided in AID, because an alternative donor can always be used. Probably everyone carries recessive genes for a few—four to eight or more—defects, so one cannot reasonably require that a donor not be a carrier of *any* defects. Some defects such as nearsightedness are not serious enough to bar someone from being a donor. If a couple is using AID to avoid transmission of a particular defect, then the donor should be screened for that trait. Beyond this, couples can work out by agreement with a physician or infertility clinic exactly what conditions a donor will be screened for.

Case 1.3 A single woman, Elaine, wants to have a child but not to get married or to engage in sexual intercourse. She attempts to receive AID, but the physician refuses. However, she learns how to do it herself using a syringe and glass jar. She has been dating a man, Fred, and he thinks they are considering marriage. He donates sperm which she uses to impregnate herself artificially. Their relationship terminates during the pregnancy. After birth of the child, Fred wants to visit the baby, but Elaine refuses to let him do so. He brings suit in court for visitation rights.[8]

This case reverses the usual situation of a sperm donor, because here the donor does want parental rights, and presumably, parental responsibilities. Ought the woman ethically to be permitted to deny him such rights? The answer should depend on the agreement made by the donor and recipient. The case ends up in court because of disagreement about the conditions of that agreement. In the end, the court gives Fred visitation rights on the ground that this was the implicit understanding.

This case also raises the issue of whether it is ethically wrong for single women to use artificial insemination to have children. Elaine was refused by a clinic, but she succeeded anyway. A number of women are like her; they would like to have a child but not to marry or to have sexual intercourse, sometimes because their sexual preferences are lesbian.

Are there any important reasons to support an ethical principle prohibiting single women from being parents? The principle of reproductive freedom does not imply that people can ethically have children whenever they want. In particular cases, it has to be balanced against other considerations such as the principle concerning risk to the unborn. Thus, concern for children can make it ethically wrong to reproduce. Is a single parent likely to be harmful to a child? Unfortunately, the answer is not perfectly clear. Suppose that statistically children with a single parent do not fare as well—emotionally, intellectually, and so on—as children with two parents. Even so, many single parents do a better job of parenting than some couples. Moreover,

[7]Curie-Cohen, "Current Practice of Artificial Insemination," p. 586.

[8]See C.M. v. C.C., 152 N.J. Super. 160, 377 A.2d 821 (Cumberland County Ct. 1977). The names in the text are invented for stylistic reasons.

many children in the United States now live in single-parent households. One can respond that most of them do still have two parents, even though they are separated or divorced. The issue here is whether a child should be brought into the world having only one social parent. There simply is no evidence that such single parents would be harmful to children. At best, one can answer only on a case-by-case basis—is this woman likely to be a competent parent? Frequently, incompetent parents are those who do not want children, but such people do not seek to have children by artificial insemination.

A further concern might attach to lesbian women. One might fear that their sexual preference would be transferred to their children. Female children might grow up hating males, and male children might grow up sexually confused. No reliable evidence exists one way or the other about such concerns. What little observational evidence there is indicates that lesbian women can be competent parents.[9] In the absence of any strong evidence that lesbians are poor parents, ethical prohibition of AID for lesbians cannot be justified. Physicians and infertility clinics need not assist individuals who will probably be incompetent or abusive parents, but that does not justify refusing lesbians as a group.

Policy Analysis

As discussed in the Introduction, questions of social policy (especially those involving political-legal control) should be kept distinct from questions of ethics. The basic policy question is whether a rational person would accept a principle for the control of conduct by the power of the state or other organization. A particular concern is with legal regulation. Will persons with rational desires and values accept a particular law for a society in which they expect to live? In answering this question, one important factor is whether effective control to achieve the purpose is possible. One of the major problems, as with the earlier prohibition of alcohol in the United States and with current laws against marijuana use, is that such laws cannot be effectively enforced, at least not without excessive loss to other values. If enforcement cannot be effective, then it is apt to waste resources and bring the law into disrepute. Another concern about the use of laws is whether they apply equally. Do they treat similar cases alike? If not, then they are discriminatory and unacceptable. We shall briefly consider a number of social policy issues about AID.

What should be the policy regarding the legitimacy of AID children and the assignment of legal parental rights? Some policy must exist, for the law must decide that people do or do not have parental rights and responsibilities, and that children are legitimate or not. Given that legal policies are necessary, there is no reason why here they should not follow general ethical principles. Husbands of women artificially inseminated by donors should have parental rights and responsibilities if and only if they gave consent for AID. Children would then be the legitimate offspring of the couple. If a wife uses AID without her husband's consent, the situation can be handled

[9]"Lesbian Couples: Should Help Extend to A.I.D.?" *Journal of Medical Ethics,* 4, no. 2 (1978), 93.

as it would be if she became pregnant by adulterous sexual intercourse—the husband is presumed to be the father unless he can prove he is not. Similarly, the parental relationships of donors would be those contractually agreed to when the donation is made, assuming the recipient also accepts those conditions.

Should the practice of artificial insemination be restricted to physicians? This is the case in a few states now, but such legislation seems unwise. As the case of Elaine (Case 1.3) makes clear, artificial insemination is a simple procedure that can be performed by almost anyone, so in practice such legislation cannot be enforced. The reasons offered for the regulation are to ensure hygienic procedures and screening of donors.[10] But it is ludicrous to seek to impose sterile procedures for artificial insemination; fairness would require the same condition for sexual intercourse, but reproduction by intercourse has occurred rather successfully without the use of rubbing alcohol! Screening might seem a better reason, but again couples reproducing by sexual intercourse do little or no screening. None of this is intended to say that physicians should not use hygienic procedures and should not screen donors; but in fairness it should not be illegal for nonphysicians to practice AID, especially a woman herself. One could end up convicting a woman for illegally getting pregnant by syringe rather than penis.

Should the law prohibit artificial insemination for single women? Enforcement would be nearly impossible. It would also be unfair, since single women can become pregnant by sexual intercourse. Besides, as discussed above, many single women are better parents than some couples. At any rate, compared to divorce and to sexual intercourse by unmarried women, no serious social consequences would result from single women who become parents by AID. Moreover, such a prohibition would violate legal principles prohibiting discrimination on the basis of marital status.[11]

Should payment to semen donors be prohibited? Statistics on blood donors indicate that more contaminated blood is obtained when donors are paid than when they are volunteers. One might expect similar results for sperm donors; in order to earn the fee, prospective donors might lie about known genetic defects in themselves or family members. Drug addicts have been known to sell sperm to get money for drugs.[12] Nevertheless, even if such a prohibition were salutary, it would be impossible to enforce generally. Women who obtain donors privately rather than through infertility clinics or physicians could easily pay without much chance of being punished. Since the concern here is with transmission of genetic defects, the real question involves what type of screening is appropriate.

Should the law require specific types of genetic screening of donors? As

[10]Jeffrey M. Shaman, "Legal Aspects of Artificial Insemination," 18 *J. Fam. L.*, 346 (1979–80); Law Reform Commission of Saskatchewan, *Tentative Proposals for a Human Artificial Insemination Act* (Saskatoon: Law Reform Commission of Saskatchewan, 1981), p. xviii.

[11]Law Reform Commission, *Tentative Proposals*, pp. 1–2; Fernando Albanese, "Artificial Insemination: Is There Movement Towards European Legislation?" in *Human Artificial Insemination and Semen Preservation*, ed. Georges David and Wendel S. Price (New York: Plenum Press, 1980), p. 481.

[12]"Sperm Donated Mainly for Money," *The Globe and Mail* (Toronto), April 24, 1981, p. 15.

noted previously, donors are commonly screened by a medical history and perhaps a blood test for Rh compatibility. Persons rationally desire to avoid transmission of genetic defects where possible. However, most couples who use natural reproduction do not engage in extensive genetic screening. Moreover, as one cannot regulate artificial insemination generally, only screening by physicians and infertility clinics could be effectively controlled. The expense of extensive screening could also put AID beyond the reach of poor people without health insurance.

Two forms of regulation appear appropriate. First, physicians providing AID should be required to conform to the standards of the profession, which certainly includes screening donors by medical history and rejecting donors known to be carriers of serious defects. Currently there is no generally accepted standard of medical practice, but perhaps health regulations should set a minimum. Second, as part of informed consent, recipients should be told what screening has been done, and what the risks of transmission of defects are; this should also be part of required disclosure in sales by sperm banks. Recipients could request specific genetic tests of donors whose sperm they receive. In short, sperm banks and physicians would be subject to civil suit for violations on the basis of negligence standards. Criminal penalties are not needed.

Should maintenance of full records be mandatory, and should they later be available to children born by AID? One reason for keeping records would be to determine whether a donor had a hidden genetic defect, and if so, not use his sperm again. This reason, however, does not justify keeping records after one has ceased to use sperm from that donor. The chief reasons for keeping records are to provide information to children.

Like many other people, AID children may desire to know their biological parents. Such a desire is emphasized in adoption situations. But is this desire a rational one? Finding out who one's genetic father is means learning his personal identity. Why would that be important? The mere knowledge does not entitle one to inheritance, other financial support, or love. What one's genetic father is or was—criminal, actor, politician, industrial worker—does not, except for certain genetic traits, determine or indicate what type of person one is or is going to become. Thus, although this desire is not necessarily irrational, if one fully understands what is involved in such information and its implications for one's own life, it probably would not be a strong desire. Much of the current interest is probably culturally conditioned (and exaggerated by the media). In addition, AID children may be significantly concerned about the possibility of inheriting a genetic disease. Such a concern certainly is rational, but fulfilling it does not require learning the donor's personal identity.

A number of reasons can be given for not requiring retention of any records that would identify donors. First, donors may have a strong desire for anonymity and may have agreed to donate only if they remain anonymous; if records of identity are not kept, anonymity is assured. Of course, if anonymity is not to be permitted, then donors in the future could not expect to remain unknown. The result might be fewer donors, or general use of frozen sperm from deceased donors. Second, the requirement to keep donor identity records can at best be effectively imposed only on physicians and infertility clinics. Individuals can practice artificial insemination privately, and it would be practically impossible to enforce such a requirement there. Third, a considerable number of children are born to married couples where the husband is not the genetic father.[13] In these situations record keeping is basically not possible; requiring it for AID by physicians and clinics is discriminatory and would affect only a few of the many children whose social fathers are not their genetic fathers. Fourth, physicians and clinics often will not know the whereabouts of a donor or whether he has developed a genetic disease. Consequently, they will not be able to learn new information that might benefit offspring. Moreover, as genetics develops, it will become possible to determine much of any individual's genetic makeup from tests performed on that individual. In short, people are likely to be able to learn more about their genetic makeup from tests performed on them than from their genetic parents. Fifth, two or more different donors are often used in a single menstrual cycle, making it difficult to say who the genetic father is. Overall, it appears that retaining records of the personal identity of donors after all children have been born from their donations is not worth the effort. It would affect only some of the many people who do not know their genetic fathers; it might discourage people from being donors; and it is not likely to produce much valuable genetic information that cannot be obtained from the individual. Indeed, the value of keeping any records for an appreciable length of time is doubtful.

Should there be policies restricting the number of times a particular donor can be used to produce a child? The primary concern here is to avoid biological incest; children from the same donor (half-siblings) might unknowingly marry or have offspring. This concern is not purely fanciful and the situation has almost occurred.[14] It also provides an additional reason in favor of keeping records. However, one must ask what the concern with incest is about. The psychological harm of sexual relations with siblings would not apply to two half-siblings from AID. Consequently, the concern must be with the genetic risks. A greater risk of transmission of genetic defects does exist. There is a one in sixteen risk of the expression of any recessive gene carried by the father. And if the same donor is used repeatedly in a community, the chance of a biologically incestuous relationship between offspring increases.

The mathematical random chance of two such half-siblings marrying is low. If one percent of the population results from AID and each donor produces ten children, there would be less than one such marriage in twenty years.[15] This possibility is not greater than that resulting from the adventures of a lothario. A number of males in any community father children by several women, unbeknownst to the husbands and children. Nonetheless,

---

[13] About 14 percent of the putative fathers of newborn black children in Detroit could not be the genetic fathers; see Curie-Cohen, "Current Practice of Artificial Insemination," p. 589. One blood test study found that in an English town, 30 percent of husbands could not be the genetic fathers of their wives' children; see E. E. Philipp, "Discussion: Moral, Social and Ethical Issues," in *Law and Ethics of A.I.D. and Embryo Transfer,* Ciba Foundation Symposium 17, new series (New York: Associated Scientific Publishers, 1973), p. 63.

[14] Hoffer, "The Legal Limbo of AID—Artificial Insemination by Donor," *Modern Medicine,* Nov. 1, 1979, p. 27, cited in Shaman, "Legal Aspects," p. 339, n. 41.

[15] Hans Moses, "Population Genetics and AID," in *Human Artificial Insemination and Semen Preservation,* ed. Georges David and Wendel S. Price (New York: Plenum Press, 1980), p. 381.

some reasonable limit upon the number of times a donor can be used seems appropriate. Institutional and professional guidelines of not using the same donor for more than ten pregnancies seem sufficient.

Surrogate Motherhood

Case 1.4 Georgia and Harold have been married for seven years. Both are intelligent, reasonably educated, and have stable jobs. Harold is thirty-two years old and Georgia is twenty-nine. For the first two years of their marriage they used contraception to avoid having children until they were on a sound financial footing. Now they own, or at least are paying for, their own home. Before they have a child, Georgia becomes ill and has to have a hysterectomy. For several months Georgia is despondent; she feels she is less a woman because she cannot have children. She wants desperately to have and raise Harold's child. One day, she reads about surrogate mothers in a women's magazine. A couple agreed to pay a woman's medical expenses if she was artificially inseminated with the man's sperm, carried the child to term, and gave it to them for adoption. Georgia wants to try the method. It is not ideal; Georgia will not bear the child for Harold, but it is the best they can do. At least Georgia can help raise Harold's child.

They go to an attorney who handles such matters. He explains the procedure to them, then sends them home to think about it. They decide to go ahead. On the next visit, the attorney provides them with information concerning three women who have been medically and psychologically screened to be surrogate mothers. Georgia and Harold are given a choice of contacting the women directly or remaining anonymous. They decide they can make a final decision only after meeting the potential surrogate mother. In the end, they select Ingrid, a divorced woman who already has a child.

Harold and Georgia agree to pay all of Ingrid's medical expenses, as well as all legal fees, life insurance, plus $10,000 to Ingrid for her time and effort in carrying the child. In return, Ingrid agrees to undergo a series of tests during pregnancy, to take care of her health, to abide by the directions of the physician, and to relinquish all rights to the child immediately upon its birth.

Ingrid does not become pregnant until the third month of inseminations. After that, the pregnancy goes normally. She meets with Georgia several times and near the end of the pregnancy she and Georgia speak over the phone each day. When the baby is delivered, Georgia and Harold are at the hospital. When the baby is released from the hospital, they take it home with them. The attorney then proceeds to file for adoption, and in a few months Georgia has adopted the baby. Harold does not have to adopt, because as Ingrid is not married, he is listed as the father on the birth certificate.

Surrogate mothering is not a widespread practice, but it does occur. Variations on the above example are possible. Perhaps the most important is that in many places, if an adoption occurs the surrogate mother cannot legally be paid, except for expenses such as medical care. If the surrogate mother is married, the adoption proceeding can be more complicated, for her husband might be legally presumed to be the father of her child. Another very common variation is for the couple never to meet the surrogate mother. Single persons rather than couples can also hire surrogate mothers. For example, a single male might want a surrogate mother to have his child. Also, a surrogate could be inseminated by donor sperm to bear a child for a single woman who cannot bear a child.

The desires or motivations for using surrogate mothers are similar to those for AID. Surrogate mothers overcome female sterility as AID overcomes male sterility. However, a surrogate mother, like Ingrid, provides not only her ovum but also her womb during gestation. Although surrogate mothering does not fulfill Georgia's desires to beget and bear a child, it does fulfill Harold's desire to beget, and both their desires to rear a child.

Ethical Analysis

A number of issues concerning surrogate motherhood are similar to those in AID, and the same principles apply to them. For example, appropriate genetic screening is typically handled in surrogate motherhood by testing as required by the requesting party (person or persons requesting a woman to be a surrogate or uterine mother). The consent of a spouse is more easily handled than in AID. If a husband had a surrogate mother impregnated without his wife's consent, she would not have to adopt. Ethically he should obtain her consent beforehand, at least if he expects to bring the child into their "family." The question of single parents also prompts the same arguments as in AID.

Surrogate motherhood raises three important ethical issues not involved in AID. Because the woman does not gestate the child, there might be important psychological consequences for her or the child that might make it wrong. Second, the consequences of the requesting party or the uterine mother not wanting to comply with some element of the agreement need to be determined. Third, the payment of a fee raises an ethical issue.

One might object to surrogate motherhood but not AID on the ground that in surrogate motherhood the child is not borne in a loving marital relationship. In AID the pregnancy occurs within the marriage; in surrogate motherhood it does not. Women who carry fetuses are much more likely than sperm donors to become emotionally attached to their offspring. A child might find it more psychologically disturbing to learn that its uterine mother gave it up for adoption than to learn that it was conceived through AID. The child might, as do some adopted children, believe that its mother rejected it because of some personal defect.

These considerations could bear on the ethical permissibility of surrogate motherhood in two distinct ways. First, it might be held that surrogate motherhood is ethically wrong simply because the gestation is not within a loving marriage. (Of course, this is not true if the surrogate is happily married.) It is difficult to see why biological gestation should be so important. During the Vietnam war, frozen semen of troops was shipped home to inseminate wives. In these cases, the couples were physically separated during gestation. Indeed, in one case the child was conceived after the father was dead. Besides, we have already seen that it is ethically acceptable for unmarried persons to have children whose gestation is not within a loving marriage.

Second, one might emphasize the possible psychological harm to the child and uterine mother (or her other children if she has them) as reasons for prohibiting surrogate motherhood. Such a concern, however, needs to be based on evidence of harm. As yet, no evidence exists. Indeed, preliminary evidence indicates that surrogate mothers do not appear to have any major psychological problems, although it is recommended that special support services be available to them.[16] Nor do their other children appear to have significant problems. Counseling might also be provided for children, should there be problems. Little reason exists to expect the psychological consequences for the child to be worse than those of adoption; indeed, they should be less. The uterine mother should know and fully understand her commitment before becoming pregnant; and the child has good reason to view the uterine mother as having performed a loving act to help others, not as simply rejecting her offspring. Consequently, psychological consequences do not provide reasons to condemn surrogate motherhood ethically.

The agreement between the uterine mother and the requesting party can break down in several ways. The uterine mother might change her mind and want an abortion; she might behave in ways that jeopardize the health of the fetus; or she might decide that she wants to keep the child, as has already happened in one case. Should the child be born with a defect, the requesting party might reject the child. Essentially, the question is how much ethical weight to assign to contractual commitments as against other considerations.

Provided the contractual requirements regarding health care are reasonable, the uterine mother's desires to engage in behaviors risking the health of the fetus do not outweigh her commitment. Indeed, it is prima facie ethically wrong to risk serious defects in an unborn child. A woman's desires to smoke or drink, for example, are not sufficient reasons to outweigh this principle, but the risks to the child may be small. Generally, an occasional drink or moderate smoking is not unethical. Here, however, the woman might also have voluntarily agreed to forgo such behaviors. The two considerations together—risk and agreement—are sufficient to make such behaviors wrong.

The two crucial problems concern a uterine mother's possible desire to have an abortion or to keep the child. Both cases involve very fundamental desires or interests of the woman—controlling her reproduction and rearing a child. As far as abortion goes, the uterine mother should have considered all the factors before entering into the agreement. Ethically, unless there is a threat to her physical or mental health, she should proceed with the pregnancy. If she does not, then she is ethically obligated to compensate the requesting party. Should she want to keep the child, then there is a conflict between the desires of the requesting party to rear the child, and those of

[16]Philip Parker, "The Psychology of Surrogate Motherhood: An Updated Report of a Longitudinal Pilot Study," presented at the Interdisciplinary Surrogate Mother Symposium, Wayne State University, Detroit, 20 November 1982 (photocopy).

the uterine mother. However, assuming the child would not be adversely affected either way, the uterine mother's promise to relinquish the child tips the scales to the requesting party.

Finally, the requesting party ought to accept the child even if it has a defect. Couples who conceive by sexual intercourse are ethically responsible for defective children. (Legally, they can relinquish their rights.) If one voluntarily undertakes to conceive a child, one is responsible for the results, just as one is responsible for the foreseeable consequences of any other voluntary action. And, as in the case of Georgia and Harold, such a risk is explicitly undertaken. If the requesting party will not accept physical possession of the child, then it ought to pay for care of the child whether that care is provided by the uterine mother or someone else, the same as for children conceived by sexual intercourse.

Probably the most controversial aspect of surrogate motherhood is the payment of a fee to the uterine mother. Two major concerns arise. First, the child appears to be bought and sold like a piece of property, but this amounts to slavery; infants are no more the property of their parents than are slaves morally property. Second, poor women might be exploited—turned into reproductive machines in order to earn money.

Although the first concern probably leads many people to consider surrogate motherhood wrong, on analysis it does not present a major objection. What is being bought and sold is not the child but the surrogate's services or the rights and responsibilities which constitute the parental role.[17] Since the bundle of parental rights does not include those of property, the child is not being treated as property. The child still has any rights vis-à-vis the parents that other children have, for example, the right not to be abused. Thus, the child is no more a slave (who lacks such rights) than other children are. With the various burdens and responsibilities of parenthood, it is unlikely that people would pay large sums of money to acquire children unless they wanted them very much. Thus, although some people might pay from improper motives and treat children badly, the chances are not great enough to condemn the whole practice. The motives of some people who have children by sexual intercourse are equally bad, but this is not a reason for condemning all reproduction by that method.

The second concern has two sides. Poor women might be exploited by especially attractive payments, and poor people might be unable to pay the going price for a surrogate mother and thus unfairly be deprived of having children by this method. Although it sounds convincing, the first consideration can be refuted upon reflection. Poor women, it is true, might be attracted by large fees to become surrogate mothers, just as other people are attracted by large fees to become lawyers or physicians. Poor, uneducated women might not have many alternatives for securing high fees. Still, this is not a reason for thinking it wrong to offer such fees. Condemning it is tantamount to accepting the following principle: Because poor, uneducated women lack other opportunities to earn large amounts of money (perhaps unjustly), they should also be denied this opportunity. Seen in this light, it

---

[17]See Lawrence A. Alexander and Lyla H. O'Driscoll, "Stork Markets: An Analysis of 'Baby-selling'," *Journal of Libertarian Studies*, 4, no. 2 (1980), 174–75.

would be unjust deprivation to deny them opportunities to be uterine mothers for a fee. Of course, this assumes that women make an informed and voluntary decision to be surrogate mothers.

The second consideration is somewhat more difficult to analyze. If prices for the services of a uterine mother are high, poor people will not be able to afford them. But, if many women decide to be surrogate mothers, the price will drop. Furthermore, not all surrogate mothers demand a fee; some do it solely to help childless people. Also, more children would probably be available for adoption by the poor. Finally, even if the prices were high and poor people could not afford them, they would be no worse off than at present. In general, one should not accept limitations on otherwise permissible activities because poor people cannot afford them, but should try to raise the income of the poor or subsidize the activities so that poor people can afford them. In short, if everyone involved voluntarily and knowingly consents to participate in surrogate motherhood and the rights of children are protected, everyone involved is better off and no one else is worse off.

Policy

Legal control over surrogate mothers is apt to be more effective than that over AID because many requesting parties will want or need a legal adoption. There are exceptions. If a single male obtains the services of a surrogate mother and is listed as the father on the birth certificate, then he has no need to adopt. At most, he needs to obtain custody of the child, and that requires only the consent of the uterine mother. Even a couple need not adopt; if the male's sperm is used, he can often be the legal father. Custody is all that is needed; the resulting family will be like many second marriages in which children are not adopted by the stepparent. In Canada, however, the father would have to go through an adoption-like process even for custody.

Just as no need was established to prohibit single females from reproducing by AID, no further reason can be given against single males becoming parents with the help of surrogate mothers. The case of single female parents would be somewhat different because they would not be genetically related to the children. However, if single women are permitted to adopt, then there is no reason to treat surrogate motherhood differently. It might be claimed that in adoption one is making the best of the situation with the child already in existence. However, there is no shortage of couples wanting to adopt, so if single parents are unacceptable, one should not let them adopt either. But of course, as noted above, some single parents are better parents than some couples. Moreover, a significant difference exists between deciding to reproduce and adoption. In adoption a child exists and placement should be based on its best interests. We do not require that decisions to reproduce be based on the best interests of the potential child. At most, we require (usually ethically rather than legally) that reproduction not be harmful to the child, for example, not lead to a defect or parental neglect and abuse. Consequently, no reasons exist to prohibit people from becoming single parents by surrogate motherhood.

Special legal problems concern enforcement of the contract between the requesting party and the uterine mother. Here social policy might justifiably depart from ethical evaluation. Historically, the law has been reluctant to require specific performance of contracted personal services, that is, make a person actually provide the services. One major reason is the difficulty of enforcement. How, for example, could the law in practice prevent a surrogate mother from smoking or drinking alcohol? Specific performance requires too great an intrusion on a uterine mother's control of her life. Consequently, the law should not require specific performance of contractual elements such as medical testing and lifestyle restrictions. As to abortion, in the United States the surrogate mother may have a Constitutional right not to be prevented from having an abortion, although that right could conceivably be contracted away. The law should treat the contract in these respects like any other contract and impose financial damages for breach, except for an abortion for the health of the uterine mother. Contracts should specify an amount for damages. To require people to perform these services is unacceptable, but it is acceptable to make them pay for the expenses and anguish others have incurred in reliance on their promises.

In one respect, specific performance might be a remedy—requiring the surrogate mother to relinquish her rights and awarding custody of the child to the requesting party. In such a case, the well-being of the child is also at stake. Indeed, given the importance of nurturing to the value of the child's entire life, the interests of the child override the desires to rear and the contractual rights of both parties. Otherwise, the child would be treated like property. Consequently, decisions of custody should be made primarily on the standard legal ground of the child's best interests, vague as it is. However, courts should be careful not to use the traditional sexist presumption that a child is better off with its natural mother. Whenever the child would be equally well off with either party, contractual obligations can determine custody in favor of the requesting party.

Another special legal concern with surrogate motherhood is the payment of a fee. The traditional reasons for prohibiting payment of fees for adoptions are to prevent baby-selling and exploitation. As we saw, these considerations are not ethically compelling for surrogate motherhood. They are no more compelling in the law. When single males do not need to adopt, they can pay fees. An unjustifiable inequality results if married males are prevented from paying fees so that their wives can legally adopt. Consequently, paying fees for the services of a surrogate mother should be legally permissible. Semen donors for artificial insemination are paid for their services, so surrogate mothers might also properly be paid for their much greater services. However, for their own protection, surrogate mothers should have separate legal counsel, and not use the same legal firm as the requesting party, as is sometimes the case now.

In Vitro Fertilization

Case 1.5 In late 1976, John and Lesley Brown consulted Dr. Patrick Steptoe. For years they had wanted to have a child, but Lesley's oviducts (small tubes that carry eggs from the ovaries to the uterus) were blocked. An earlier operation to try to remove the blockage had been unsuccessful. A few months later Dr. Steptoe, using a laparoscope (a small viewing instrument inserted into the abdomen), examined Lesley's ovaries and found them covered with adhesions. In a subsequent operation he removed much of this scar tissue. By then it was August 1977.

That November, just before Lesley would have ovulated naturally, Dr. Steptoe again performed a laparoscopy. This time, he removed a ripe ovum or egg from an ovary a few hours before it normally would have left. Dr. Robert Edwards then placed the ovum in a laboratory dish with sperm from John. One of the sperm fertilized the ovum, and the resulting embryo was cultured for two and a half days. Late at night, the embryo was taken into a syringe, and Dr. Steptoe inserted it through the cervix into Lesley's uterus.

Lesley became pregnant. Later, tests were performed and the fetus was found to be free of any determinable genetic problems. Although the fetal growth lagged behind normal and Lesley developed toxemia, the pregnancy continued. On the evening of July 25, 1978, Dr. Steptoe delivered a baby girl—Louise Joy Brown—by cesarean section. She was the world's first "test-tube baby."

The method of conception just described involves *in vitro* fertilization (*in vitro* meaning in glass—a laboratory dish or test tube) and embryo transfer, that is, transferring the embryo from the laboratory dish to the womb. Since the birth of Louise Brown, a number of other children have been conceived by this technique in half a dozen or more countries, and the number of clinics practicing the technique is growing rapidly. In 1982, over thirty clinics were established in the United States alone. The technique, at least so far, is not as effective as natural conception. Only about ten out of one hundred women from whom ova are obtained will have a live birth, whereas about thirty-one of one hundred women who have sexual intercourse during their fertile time in a month have a live birth.[18] However, the success rate of *in vitro* fertilization is increasing; at the same time probably 50 percent of all naturally fertilized ova fail to result in recognizable pregnancies.

In vitro fertilization with embryo transfer normally uses the sperm and ova of a married couple, and the embryo is implanted in the wife. However, all sorts of variations are possible, at least one of which has been used. The sperm or ovum or both could be donated. (Donated sperm can be used for single women.) The gestating mother need not be the genetic mother, nor the social father the genetic father. Indeed, up to five different "parents" could be involved: two people could donate sperm and an ovum, the embryo could gestate in the uterus of a second woman, and an entirely different man and woman rear the child.

In vitro fertilization (IVF) is most frequently used to overcome female infertility. In the standard case, as with Louise Brown, the genetic and social father are the same, as are the genetic, uterine, and social mother. Thus, the desires of a couple to beget, bear, and rear are all fulfilled. A possible

---

[18]John D. Biggers, "In Vitro Fertilization and Embryo Transfer in Human Beings," *New England J. Med.*, 304, no. 6 (1981), 339.

variation, say, if the woman has had a hysterectomy but still has functioning ovaries, is to use the sperm and ovum of the couple but have another woman gestate the child. This is comparable to surrogate motherhood as discussed above, except that the surrogate is not the genetic mother. As the desires for begetting, bearing, and rearing are all fulfilled in the standard case, in this respect the argument for IVF is stronger than for AID or surrogate motherhood.

Ethical Analysis

Many arguments have been offered at one time or another against the ethical permissibility of IVF. A number of them have already been discussed in connection with AID and surrogate motherhood. One might object to the biological separation of a loving sexual act and reproduction, or to the use of IVF for single parents. One might object that people could bear or rear children to whom they were not genetically related. Each of these objections was considered with respect to AID or surrogate motherhood and rejected. Consequently, the only arguments against IVF that need to be examined are those that pertain to the technique itself.

Many people have questioned the safety of IVF. The concern is that the manipulations of the sperm, ovum, and embryo might cause defects, resulting in more abnormal children than intercourse. The evidence is now fairly strong that IVF does not involve a significant increase in genetic defects, although about three thousand births will be needed to establish that reliably. Embryos appear to be quite resistant to damage, and if they are damaged are likely to die. About 5 percent of all infants are born with some genetic or congenital defect. Approximately 50 percent of spontaneous abortions and failures to implant, especially during early pregnancy, are due to genetic defects. Consequently, IVF embryos with chromosomal defects are apt to be naturally aborted. Little evidence exists of increased risk of other defects.[19] The additional risks are probably less than the added risks for a woman in her late thirties having a child by normal intercourse.

Some people have objected that IVF amounts to unethical nontherapeutic experimentation on unborn children without their consent.[20] Although at present IVF should perhaps still be classified as an experimental procedure, it is less clear that the procedure is nontherapeutic. The resulting child receives the benefit of life and any value life contains. Were the procedure not performed, the child would not exist. Moreover, it is incoherent to require the consent of a nonexistent person. Were this an ethical requirement, then it would be unethical to use any techniques, such as surgery or hormones, to overcome infertility, for any such technique might cause damage to a child. An ethical principle prohibiting any experimentation in conception, no matter how small the risks, is not acceptable.

Nonetheless, some people contend that one should not perform IVF if its risks are greater than those of conception by intercourse. And we sug-

[19]Biggers, "In Vitro Fertilization," p. 341.

[20]See, for example, Paul Ramsey, "Shall We 'Reproduce'?" *JAMA,* 220, no. 10 (1972), 1346–50, and 220, no. 11 (1972), 1480–85.

gested earlier that it is wrong to take substantial risks of significant defects in unborn children. One problem is determining what constitutes a normal conception and thus normal risk. The risks in IVF are almost certainly less than those in many conceptions, such as those by couples at increased risk for having a child with a defect because of a family history of a defect. Somewhat greater risks of defect than in normal conceptions are probably justifiable to overcome infertility. Even if they are not, the requirement of normal risks is probably met.

In some clinics, most of the women are in their late thirties and thus at increased risk for having children with genetic defects. Moreover, almost all these women refuse amniocentesis to test for defects because it slightly increases the chances of a spontaneous abortion. They do not want to risk the loss of a fetus after so much effort to become pregnant. Still, even with a slight increase of risk of defect due to IVF, the risk of defect is much less than that of many women reproducing by sexual intercourse.

Another objection to IVF is that it involves the destruction of nascent human life—embryos or fetuses. This argument has two versions. The more common one is that extra embryos will be produced and destroyed rather than implanted.[21] The less common one is that, as with Lesley Brown, prenatal diagnosis will be performed and some fetuses will be aborted because they have defects. Both versions assume that the previable embryo or fetus is protectable human life. The second version also assumes that abortion of defective fetuses is wrong. It is not an argument against IVF but against prenatal diagnosis and abortion, because it applies equally well to fetuses conceived by sexual intercourse. And as just noted, most older women reject amniocentesis.

The first version of the argument does not assume that only defective embryos will be discarded. However, its force depends on the technique used. The method used by Drs. Steptoe and Edwards for Lesley Brown did not involve discarding any embryos in the actual procedure, although some were destroyed in earlier experiments. Only one ovum was recovered and fertilized per menstrual cycle, and that embryo was tranferred. However, if no pregnancy results, one must perform laparoscopy again in order to recover another ovum. Given the low rates of live birth per laparoscopy, repeated laparoscopies involving general anesthesia are often required before a woman becomes pregnant, and some never do. To avoid repeated laparoscopies, another technique is to use drugs to produce superovulation and try to recover several ripe ova. Some practitioners fertilize and transfer two or more embryos in order to increase the chances of implantation. Some are also freezing some embryos for later use, and pregnancy has been achieved with such an embryo. In at least one clinic, most women donate extra ova to women from whom ova cannot be obtained. Alternatively, one ovum at a time can be fertilized and transferred; other ova might be frozen for later use if needed. (So far, reliable techniques for freezing ova have not been developed.) Even if it were wrong to discard nondefective human embryos, none of these techniques needs to involve discarding them. Of course, some embryos might be used for experimentation or destroyed.

[21]See, for example, Raymond A. Belliotti, "Morality and *In Vitro* Fertilization," *Bioethics Quarterly*, 2, no. 1 (Spring 1980), 6–19.

Thus, this objection does not show that all IVF is wrong. At the best, it could constitute an objection to producing embryos that were not to be implanted. In Chapter 4 it is argued that embryos at this stage are not protectable human life.

The freezing of human embryos does not raise any ethical objections not already considered. It could involve a question of safety, but evidence with freezing animal embryos suggests that it is safe. No new ethical principle is involved. Also, extra frozen embryos might be discarded, but they need not be; they could be transferred to other women. Consent of embryos is no more a rational requirement here than it is for their creation.

Policy Analysis

IVF can be effectively regulated because, unlike artificial insemination, it requires the involvement of medical practitioners. Nonetheless, no reasons exist for any special regulation of IVF. One can assume that it will be controlled by the usual legal standards of medical practice with respect to negligence, informed consent, and so on. These should cover aspects of the technique involving the manipulation of the ova, sperm, and embryos such as sterile procedures, and so forth. In the standard case, as with Louise Brown, no issues of legitimacy or adoption arise. In the nonstandard types of situations that are possible, the considerations are no different than for AID or surrogate motherhood or a combination of them. The destruction of embryos would be covered by abortion laws (to be considered later). One might need a regulation requiring the consent of women or parents to use ova or embryos not to be implanted in them. Other than that, no regulations are needed for IVF that are not also needed for AID or surrogate motherhood.

At this point, several common threads in the discussion of AID, surrogate motherhood, and IVF should be noted. First, many suggested restrictions on the use of these methods would prohibit infertile people doing what others do by sexual intercourse. Examples are the concerns for single parents, genetic risk, sterile procedures, and record keeping. Thus, many of the fears concern matters which are not likely to be any worse than conception as it has always occurred. Although not all past practices of conception are good, it is unjust to impose restrictions on infertile people when their risks are no worse than those of ordinary conception. Second, many matters cannot be effectively regulated. Artificial insemination is so simple that almost anyone can do it. Indeed, in some places artificial insemination of humans is performed with turkey basters, and the children are called "basting babies."[22]

Third, a strong motive for use of these techniques is to beget genetic offspring. A desire to beget for its own sake, we saw, is probably irrational. Although the desire for genetic offspring per se has not been accorded weight, these various techniques for fulfilling that desire have been found ethically permissible. The reason, however, has been instrumental—to fulfill the desire to rear children. With modern contraceptive techniques, in

---

[22]Christopher Reed, " 'Turkey-Baster Babies' Kept Secret in Lesbian World," *The Globe and Mail* (Toronto), August 29, 1980, p. 11.

creased abortion, and the decision of most pregnant single women to rear their children, few infants are available for adoption, at least in comparison to the demand resulting from the fact that almost one-sixth of married couples are infertile. There are older children, handicapped children, and children in the third world available for adoption, although it is sometimes difficult to adopt foreign children. Moreover, it would be unfair to make infertile couples pass up the joys of rearing infants or suffer the burdens of rearing handicapped children. Nor is it desirable to revert to the previous situation in which many women bore children they did not want. If all infertile couples had children, population growth would increase significantly, but population size can be controlled by limiting everyone's opportunity to have children rather than simply depriving infertile couples of the opportunity to rear children because of a condition for which they are often not responsible.

BIBLIOGRAPHY

BIGGERS, JOHN D. "In Vitro Fertilization and Embryo Transfer in Human Beings," *New England Journal of Medicine,* 304, no. 6 (Feb. 5, 1981), 336–41.

CURIE-COHEN, MARTIN; LUTTRELL, LESLEIGH; and SHAPIRO, SANDER "Current Practice of Artificial Insemination by Donor in the United States," *New England Journal of Medicine,* 300, no. 11 (March 15, 1979), 585–90.

DAVID, GEORGES; and PRICE, WENDEL S., eds. *Human Artificial Insemination and Semen Preservation.* New York: Plenum Press, 1980.

EDWARDS, ROBERT; and STEPTOE, PATRICK *A Matter of Life: The Story of a Medical Breakthrough.* London: Hutchinson, 1980.

GROBSTEIN, CLIFFORD *From Chance to Purpose: An Appraisal of External Human Fertilization.* Reading, Mass.: Advanced Book Program, Addison-Wesley Publishing Company, 1981.

HOLMES, HELEN B.; HOSKINS, BETTY B.; and GROSS, MICHAEL, eds. *The Custom-Made Child? Women-Centered Perspectives.* Clifton, N.J.: The Humana Press, Inc., 1981.

KEANE, NOEL P.; with BREO, DENNIS L. *The Surrogate Mother.* New York: Everest House Publishers, 1981.

SNOWDEN, R.; and MITCHELL, G.D. *The Artificial Family: A Consideration of Artificial Insemination by Donor.* London: George Allen & Unwin, 1981.

WALTERS, LEROY "Human in Vitro Fertilization: A Review of the Ethical Literature," *The Hastings Center Report,* 9, no. 4 (August 1979), 23–43.

WALTERS, WILLIAM; and SINGER, PETER, eds. *Test-Tube Babies: A Guide to Moral Questions, Present Technologies and Future Possibilities.* Melbourne: Oxford University Press, 1982.

CHAPTER 2

Genetic Choice

The last chapter outlined methods by which individuals and couples can have children genetically related to them. This chapter considers issues raised by methods developed in the last two decades that provide people some choice of the genetic features of their children. For the most part, these methods enable people to choose not to have children with certain features.

Three types of methods of genetic choice are available. One type enables people to increase the chances of having a child of a specific sex. Another type, carrier screening, enables people to determine whether they are likely to transmit deleterious genetic features to offspring. The third type, prenatal diagnosis, can be used to determine whether a fetus has some specific characteristic and then abort it if that is desirable. Not all the conditions that can be detected by prenatal diagnosis are genetic; some of them result from drugs, maternal illness, or other causes.

Sex Preselection

Case 2.1 Jeremiah and Katharine have two daughters, ages six and nine. Katharine is thirty-four years old. Jeremiah would like to have a son; indeed, he wants one very much. Katharine would like another child but does not especially care whether it is a boy or girl. However, she does not want to have more than one more child, and plans to be sterilized after the birth of the next child, whether Jeremiah likes it or not. The risks of having a child with Down syndrome are increasing as Katharine gets older; besides, she would like to go back to nursing, which she gave up when their older daughter was born.

Jeremiah reads a newspaper story describing a patented process that makes it possible to select with considerable accuracy the sex of a child at conception. The process involves taking semen from the husband and separating the male-determining sperm from the female determining sperm. The process destroys most of the female-determining sperm. Physicians at the clinic then artifically inseminate the woman with the male sperm. This process cannot be used to produce females, but Jeremiah is only interested in having a boy. Katharine agrees to the treatment; after the third month, she is pregnant. Jeremiah is joyous, because he is sure that this time he will have a son. Now and then, though, Katharine notices him sitting quietly with a worried look. She finally asks him what is wrong, and he says that he sometimes has doubts that this child will be a son, and he does not know what he will do if it is not.

In recent years, several methods in addition to the one just described have been developed to increase the chances of conceiving a child of a particular sex.[1] One technique involves injecting the woman with antibodies against male- or female-determining sperm. Animal sperm have been separated by using a medium of varying viscosity. Two methods that do not involve medical intervention have been suggested. One is to time intercourse to occur two days before ovulation in order to have a girl, or at ovulation for a boy. Another technique recommends a different timing, a vinegar douche, shallow penetration, and no female orgasm in order to have a girl; and opposite conditions for a boy. These two methods have not been well established; indeed, they recommend contrary timing of intercourse. A more accurate method, which is not yet possible, would be to ascertain the sex of embryos in IVF before transfer. Existing methods are not as accurate as IVF would be; at best, they increase the probability of a child being of one sex or another.

One rather different method for reliably determining the sex of the fetus now exists: prenatal diagnosis. At about sixteen weeks, amniotic fluid is withdrawn from the womb, fetal cells are cultured, and the sex is determined by chromosomal analysis. Some new techniques of recovering fetal cells may allow this procedure to be performed at an earlier date. To ensure the desired sex of the child, a woman must abort a fetus of the unwanted sex.

Sex Preference

Considerable evidence exists that many men and women, like Jeremiah, desire male children. Indeed, many prefer to have a male child first, and then a female. But is it rational to desire a child of a particular sex? A preference for one sex over the other, for its own sake, is simply sexism. It implies that one sex is intrinsically more valuable than another, but good reasons can be and have been given against this view by many authors, so such a desire is irrational.

---

[1]For more details, see M. Ruth Netwig, "Technical Aspects of Sex Preselection," in *The Custom-Made Child? Women-Centered Perspectives,* ed. Helen B. Holmes, Betty B. Hoskins, and Michael Gross (Clifton, N.J.: The Humana Press, Inc., 1981), pp. 181–86.

Most people would not admit to such a pure sex preference but claim that the desire for a child of a particular sex is instrumental to fulfilling other desires. However, there are strong reasons for believing that many of the most common instrumental reasons are unsound and probably mask an irrational sexism. Reasons often given in the past for instrumentally preferring children of one sex (particularly males) are to inherit, to carry on the family name, and to have workers. But none of these reasons are relevant in the modern Western world. Today, male and female children inherit equally. Females can carry on the family name if they want; they need not change their names when they marry. Few jobs exist that women cannot fulfill as well as men (and of course they are generally better than men at some jobs).

One might reply that someone like Jeremiah need not be sexist or irrational to want a boy. He has two daughters, and he would simply like to have a boy as well. Had he had two boys, he might have wanted a girl. But why would two daughters and one son be preferable to three daughters? Someone like Jeremiah might respond that he would like a son so that he could have certain pleasures in child rearing—such as fishing and playing ball with him. But that too is probably a sexist assumption. As the father of two daughters, I have fished and played ball with them, watched my daughter play on a ball team, and gone camping and hiking with them, as well as cooked, cleaned house, done laundry, and engaged in various other so-called women's activities with them.

There may be some activities that are strongly sex-related in that members of one sex are generally better at them than members of the other sex. For example, perhaps most women have a greater aptitude for ballet than men. Recognition of such differences in role aptitude is not sexist, but the assumption that no members of the other sex can perform the same roles well or that one set of such roles is preferable to the other is sexist. Thus, a desire to have a male (female) child because of a preference for one set of "sex-linked" roles is sexist. Nor can one argue that variety is desired. Were children allowed to develop freely their own interests and talents, children of the same sex would probably exhibit as much diversity as children of opposite sexes.

Consequently, an instrumental preference for a child of one sex or the other is also often irrational. However, in some cases it is reasonable to desire a child of one sex rather than another for instrumental reasons. Undoubtedly, the most serious reason concerns X-linked genetic diseases, such as hemophilia. Only males exhibit the disease; females can only be carriers. Thus, if a woman is a carrier of such a disease, it would be rational to desire female children. Ironically, this is not the sex preference most people express. In this case, sexism is not involved. The preference here is not for a female child, but for a healthy child, and a female has a significantly better chance of being healthy.

Ethical Analysis

We can assume that sexism is wrong. Arguments to this effect have been offered by many authors, and the history of sexism clearly shows the misery and unfortunate consequences it has wrought. Nonetheless, sexism is still prevalent in society. That sex preselection on the basis of intrinsic and most instrumental sex preference expresses an unethical sexist attitude is sufficient for holding that it is wrong. Its practice would probably reinforce sexist attitudes both in those who practice it and in others.

Two other general social consequences are often thought likely to result from sex preselection. First, evidence exists that most people who want a child of each sex prefer to have a male first, and that first-born children are apt to achieve more than later-born children.[2] If couples used sex preselection to have a male child first, and males were thus on average better social achievers than females, this would tend to reinforce sexist attitudes. Second, if sex preselection resulted in more males than females, the sex imbalance could have undesirable social consequences, such as insufficient mates. There might be good results as well. Population growth might decrease, because people often have more children in an attempt to have some of each sex. A better balance of male/female companionship among the elderly might result. The elderly population is now disproportionately female since women live longer than men; were there considerably more males than females born, the elderly population would be more evenly balanced between the sexes. Younger women would be in short supply and might have more social opportunities. (Of course, more younger men might then lack mates and be lonely.) However, most of these projections about the consequences of a sex imbalance are mere speculation. They are not well enough founded to support an ethical principle.

In sum, sex preselection on the basis of intrinsic sex preference is always wrong, and so is most sex preselection on the basis of instrumental sex preference. One should accept an ethical principle condemning sex preselection as the expression of irrational desires and as reinforcing sexism in society. Unlike the irrational desire for genetic offspring, these irrational desires might have further untoward consequences if people act on them. However, sex preselection for clearly rational instrumental reasons, for example, to avoid offspring with sex-linked genetic diseases, constitutes an ethically permissible and desirable exception. Jeremiah's intrinsic desire for a son is the expression of a sexist attitude, and he and Katharine are ethically wrong to try to have a son.

Policy Analysis

Although most sex preselection is ethically wrong, policies to prevent its practice are not acceptable. Laws to prohibit sexism are justifiable in many areas, but sex preselection presents special problems. It would be impossible to enforce such a prohibition in practice if timing methods were effective. Any effort to prevent the use of timing methods would involve an unacceptable governmental intrusion into people's private lives. The best

---

[2]Roberta Steinbacher, "Futuristic Implications of Sex Preselection," in *The Custom-Made Child? Women-Centered Perspectives,* ed. Helen B. Holmes, Betty B. Hoskins, and Michael Gross (Clifton, N.J.: The Humana Press, Inc., 1981), p. 188.

that could be done would be to prohibit the use of artificial insemination techniques for sex preselection by fertility clinics and others. Such a step would not effectively prevent such sex preselection, because people would lie about their reasons or an underground business would develop, so it would be pointless to restrict fertility clinics.

Should a sex imbalance result and the consequences be highly undesirable, then some social policy might be necessary and possible. The policy would not consist in prohibiting sex preselection, but in encouraging it! Incentives, such as extra tax deductions, could be offered for having children of a particular sex, or for having them first. Such policies might also reinforce sexism and would be acceptable only if the consequences of unfettered sex preselection were quite bad. Indeed, it might be wise not to accept them even then but merely to increase efforts at educating people not to be sexists.

Regardless of the ethics of abortion, the use of prenatal diagnosis and abortion for most sex selection is ethically wrong simply as sex preselection. However, that does not provide a reason for a policy against its use or withholding information about the sex of the fetus after amniocentesis. People may also simply be curious about the fetus's sex.

Carrier Screening

Case 2.2 Louis and Miriam are in their early twenties. They have been married about a year but have not yet had any children. Both want to have their life together fairly well-adjusted before taking on parental responsibilities. They hear about a program at a clinic in their city to screen Jewish couples for carrier status of the recessive gene for Tay-Sachs disease. Miriam is especially concerned about it, because a friend of hers has recently given birth to a child with Tay-Sachs. The child faces a general neurological deterioration and almost certain death before school age. Her friend is going through emotional turmoil. Louis is less enthusiastic about having the tests. "After all," he says, "the disease results from recessive genes, so there is no chance of a child of ours having the defect unless both of us are carriers. Even then, the odds are only one in four. Why not simply have prenatal diagnosis done during pregnancy to determine whether the fetus has the disease? Even if both of us are carriers, we could go ahead and conceive and use prenatal diagnosis to find out if the baby is normal."

This case concerns one of the usual forms of carrier screening, that for a recessive autosomal (non-sex chromosomal) gene which is rare but more frequently found in a specific population. For recessive conditions, both parents must be carriers before there is a chance a child will have the condition. That is, to have a recessive disease, a child must inherit an affected gene from each parent. In this case, Tay-Sachs is found with a much higher frequency among Ashkenazi Jews—those from Eastern Europe— than others. A slightly more prevalent form of carrier screening is for defects in blood—sickle cell anemia among blacks, and beta-thalassemia among people of Mediterranean origin. Most carrier screening is relatively inexpensive and accurate and involves analysis of a small blood sample. Carrier testing is possible for a few other genetic conditions, and the number continues to grow. A few conditions are caused by dominant genes; with them, only one parent need be a carrier, but that parent will also suffer from the defect or disease. Most dominant disorders are detected in spontaneous mutants.

Value Analysis

Louis's and Miriam's differing attitudes towards carrier screening center on the value of the knowledge that will be gained. The primary outcome of genetic testing is knowledge—knowing whether a person is a carrier or has a condition. Knowledge can be desired either intrinsically or instrumentally. When knowledge is intrinsically valued, a person simply wants to know something for its own sake, out of curiosity. When knowledge is desired instrumentally, it is valued because of its consequences, usually because it enables one to take some action.

Information obtainable from genetic screening is primarily of instrumental value. Some people may simply be curious about their genetic constitution, but that is not the usual reason for having the tests. People desire knowledge about carrier status in order to relieve their anxiety about having a child with a defect, and to enable them to take action to avoid having such a child. When tests are done to find out whether a newborn or adult actually has a disease, the people involved desire the knowledge in order to treat or ameliorate the condition. Sometimes the fear of finding out about a disease may be greater than any alleviation of anxiety. For example, Huntington disease results from a dominant gene and does not become manifest until later in life, usually between the ages of thirty and fifty. The disease involves progressive mental deterioration and uncontrollable physical movements. Woody Guthrie, the musician, died of it. The worry and anxiety of knowing that one has such a disease can be overwhelming, and the suicide rate amongst people who have it is high. Many people would rather not know whether or not they have it. The same may be true of some carrier screening, for some people have a lower self-image when they discover they are carriers. Thus, the bad consequences of genetic information can sometimes outweigh the good ones, and the information is not then instrumentally valuable.

The desire for genetic information is rational because it is surely rational to want to avoid having a child with a defect. One aspect of that desire is to avoid begetting (conceiving) a child with a significant handicap. Generally, a significant handicap is one that decreases the value of life to the person who lives it. The life of a child with a handicap can be of value but it is still rational to desire not to conceive such a child. Handicaps are by definition undesirable characteristics, and it is rational to avoid them. One might object that one also avoids the existence of the person, not merely the handicap. Yet, it is precisely the fact that no person exists that makes it quite rational to avoid begetting such a person. One would not, except under the most unusual circumstances, make a radio using a defective speaker even if that radio would have some value. Another aspect of the desire to avoid begetting a child with a significant handicap is to avoid the suffering of oneself and others. Handicapped children place greater burdens on their parents and siblings in terms of time, effort, and financial resources than do normal children.

Another relevant value pertains to risk taking. With recessive traits, one out of four children will have the deleterious disease. With dominant traits, one out of two children of an affected parent will have it. Other conditions have varying degrees of risk. Thus, attitudes about risk are important for making decisions. Unfortunately, no known method exists for showing that an attitude toward risk is rational or irrational. Some people are gamblers and risk-takers while others are cautious. No evidence exists that people would generally adopt one attitude rather than another were they fully informed of the facts. However, even if attitudes towards risk can rationally vary, they are not equally acceptable when the well-being of others depends on the decision. It may be reasonable to take significant risks with one's own life, for example, by riding a motorcycle, but it is unreasonable or ethically inappropriate to take significant risks with another person's life.

Ethical Analysis

Suppose Miriam talks Louis into going to the clinic to find out more about the test for Tay-Sachs. What information should Louis obtain and evaluate in order to give his informed consent to the procedure? This question is quite important in programs that involve mass screening; large-scale programs are apt to process people routinely without adequately explaining matters to them.

The point of having the test is to gain information. If Louis is to decide whether that information is worthwhile, he needs to be informed of all the relevant facts. How much will the tests cost? Sometimes the information obtainable is not worth the expense of obtaining it. Another important question is, What precisely does the procedure entail? Louis also needs to know what he can do with the test results. As such knowledge is only instrumentally valuable, he needs to know what options the information gives him. In the case of Tay-Sachs, as Louis already knows, if both he and Miriam are carriers, prenatal diagnosis can be performed to determine whether a fetus actually has the disease. Another option would be to use artificial insemination by a noncarrier donor or to use a noncarrier surrogate mother. Louis should also want to know how bad the disease is, as well as the chances that someone of his background is a carrier. In short, Louis needs to be advised of the chances that he is a carrier, the nature of the test, the nature of the disease, and all the available options for action should both he and Miriam be carriers. With less than this information, he could not make a rational decision whether or not to have the test.

It might be argued that Louis has a duty to undergo the test, that he has a duty to discover whether he is at risk of having a child with a severe genetic disease or defect. After all, his ignorance could result in the birth of a child with a serious handicap; the child would suffer the consequences of Louis's action more than Louis.

Whether Louis has a duty to have the test depends on whether he and Miriam would have a duty not to have an affected child if it were revealed that both are carriers. If they would not have such a duty, they do not have a duty to find out that they are carriers and at risk of having such a child. Two factors are relevant to whether carriers have a duty to avoid having an affected child—the value of the life to the child and the effects of its life on others. Both of these factors must then be considered in light of variable risks of having an affected child.

The principle of avoiding risk to the unborn is that it is prima facie wrong to take a substantial risk of a significant defect or handicap to an unborn child. A number of reasons support this principle. First, since the child does not exist, failure to reproduce does not harm it, and as we saw in the previous chapter, there is no duty to reproduce. Second, such a handicapped individual would lack an equal opportunity with others in society. For their own interests, parents would have deliberately brought into existence a person lacking equality of opportunity. Third, if the handicap would be so severe that life would not be of value to the individual, misery would have been inflicted on that person. Consequently, while other considerations might outweigh the prima facie wrongness of risking a significant handicap that would still leave life of value, nothing short of averting a large-scale disaster could justify bringing into existence someone whose life was of no value to that person.

The principle regarding risk to the unborn deliberately does not specify degrees of risk and handicap, only that they be substantial and significant. The two considerations must be balanced against one another. The greater the handicap, the less the risk should be; and vice versa. At this point, what makes life valuable, and thus what constitutes a significant handicap, is not fully specified. As we shall see in Chapter 5 where that issue is considered in detail, the crucial elements of a valuable life are pleasant experiences and the fulfillment of interests, both of which can be detrimentally affected by pain or lack of physical or mental abilities.

The principle regarding risk to the unborn has been justified solely by consequences for the child. However, effects on others, primarily the parents and siblings, are also relevant. The principle regarding burdens to others states that the burdens a child's life will place on others constitute an ethically relevant reason not to bring an unborn child into existence. In deciding whether to reproduce, couples should consider whether they would enjoy raising a child, as well as possible harmful effects on existing siblings. Since there is no duty to reproduce and the unborn child does not exist, it would not be harmed by not being brought into existence; but existing people might be. Thus, even if the child's life might be of value to it, the burden to others is a relevant reason for not reproducing.

Case 2.3 Nathaniel and Olive are very much in love. A year or so after their marriage, they consider having a child. However, in their situation, they think it best to talk to a genetic counselor first. Both have mildly expressed sickle cell disease, but they lead reasonably normal lives and their few attacks are under control.

The counselor tells them that pregnancy for a woman with sickle cell disease is rather risky. About half of such pregnancies result in spontaneous abortion or stillbirth, and the maternal death rate is very high.[3] Nathaniel and Olive are quite lucky that their sickle cell anemia is not severe. Ten percent of people born with the disease die by the age of ten, and many others live with great pain and are severely handicapped. Given that both of them have the disease, each of their children is also certain to have it.

This case presents an issue of risk taking. Unlike the problem of Louis and Miriam where the risk is whether a child will have the disease, in this case the risk pertains to the severity of the disease. For carriers of recessive conditions (like Louis and Miriam), the risk is one in four that their children will have the disease, and often this cannot be determined by prenatal diagnosis. The ethical questions in all of these cases are whether the principle regarding risk to the unborn applies, and whether other reasons for having a child outweigh it if it does.

In the case of Nathaniel and Olive, the principle clearly applies; a child of theirs is certain to have a life-threatening disease. The question is whether good reasons exist that outweigh the prima facie wrongness of their begetting a child together. Couples like Nathaniel and Olive may consider taking such a risk to have a child. One must here distinguish the desires to have genetic offspring, to bear offspring, and to rear them. As we have seen, the desire to beget offspring for its own sake is not rational. It is the only desire that need be frustrated if Nathaniel and Olive are to have a child without this risk of defect. If Olive were artificially inseminated with the sperm of a noncarrier donor, she could bear a child and they could both rear it. She would even have begotten the child, but not with Nathaniel. Similarly, Nathaniel could beget a child by a noncarrier surrogate mother without risk of sickle cell disease. He could even beget by a noncarrier ovum and have the embryo transferred to Olive. Consequently, only the couple's desire to beget a child with each other supports reproduction in the usual manner. As a subclass of the desire to have genetic offspring, the desire to have genetic offspring with a specific person is also irrational. It surely does not override the principle of avoiding risk to the unborn. Thus, the risk is not one that may ethically be taken.

In general, then, the desire for genetic offspring cannot override the principle of avoiding risk to the unborn. It is not, however, always clear that the principle of risk applies. Suppose a couple is at risk of having a child with a disease like galactosemia, which can result in cataracts, mental retardation, and digestive disorders. The effects of galactosemia can be controlled by diet, primarily by avoiding milk and milk products, but this can cause considerable difficulty for parents, especially in preparing meals for a

---

[3]Robert M. Veatch, *Case Studies in Medical Ethics* (Cambridge, Mass.: Harvard University Press, 1977), p. 182.

large family. With treatment, such a disease does not result in significant handicap to the individual, although it is a significant bother. Thus, the principle of risk to the unborn does not pertain, or at least has little weight. However, couples might decide not to risk such a child because of the burdens to them.

Another ethical issue that arises in carrier screening concerns confidentiality. Suppose Louis were tested and found to be a carrier of Tay-Sachs. Then each of his siblings has a 50 percent chance of being a carrier as well. Ethically, it seems clear, Louis should inform his brothers and sisters that they should also be tested. Suppose, though, he refuses to do so. May a physician suggest screening to the siblings without Louis's consent? One might suggest that his brothers and sisters need never know that Louis is a carrier; Louis's physician could simply tell them that they should be screened. But that would not work. Either Louis's siblings would know it was his doctor or they would ask why the doctor thought they should be screened. The same problem would arise were the information given to their family physicians, supposing the testing center could find out who the doctors were.

The ethical conflict is between Louis's claim to confidentiality and his siblings' claim to have information important to them. The two values must be weighed. To do so, one must clarify the situation and consider the two values or desires as affecting oneself. Louis's fear of disclosure is irrational; being a carrier does not significantly affect his health, and he is not at fault for being a carrier. Even if the claim of confidentiality is weighted heavily, in this situation the value of the information is greater than that of confidentiality. Consequently, an acceptable principle of confidentiality would allow an exception for such a case. But the exception would extend only to Louis's siblings, who should ethically keep the information confidential.

A final difficulty that arises from carrier screening pertains to truth telling. Sometimes carrier screening is not performed until after the birth of an affected child. In that case, carrier screening might indicate that the putative father is not the genetic father. Should the counselor tell the man that he is not a carrier and so there is no risk in a subsequent conception? This would clearly indicate that he was not the father. Some counselors confronted with this situation lie and say that the defect was due to a spontaneous mutation so that there is no risk in a subsequent pregnancy.[4]

Although this type of situation cannot be avoided, the ethical situation can be clarified in advance. The purpose of screening is to obtain information, and prior to the screening the putative father should be told what types of information might be obtained. Prior to consent, he should be advised that information of nonpaternity might be discovered. At that point, he can decide whether he wishes to risk finding out that information. Although a child might suffer should a putative father discover he was not the biological father and legally contest his paternity and obligation to support, this consideration is not stronger for handicapped than for normal children. Granted, the burden on a handicapped child may be greater than on a normal one, but the burden on the putative father is also greater, both emotionally and financially. Securing the putative father's consent beforehand will not make the

[4]"Genetic Screening," *Encyclopedia of Bioethics* (1978), 2, 571.

discovery any easier for him or the child, and will probably make his decision to be tested more difficult, but it clarifies the duty of the physician to inform.

Policy Analysis

The primary policy issue in carrier screening concerns legally compulsory screening. Most mandatory screening is for treatable diseases in infants, but in the early 1970s a number of states enacted laws requiring all blacks to be screened for carrier status for sickle cell disease. Sometimes the legislatures were probably confused as to what they were requiring, thinking that the tests were for the disease rather than the carrier state. Are there circumstances in which mandatory screening is acceptable?

Two related reasons might support compulsory screening for carrier status. (1) Screening might decrease the number of children born with handicapping diseases. (2) This decrease might save public funds for the care of handicapped individuals. Mandatory carrier screening will not contribute significantly to either goal. Both of these possible benefits depend on people avoiding birth of handicapped children. Screening itself only provides information enabling people to avoid giving birth to such children. At a minimum, one would also have to ensure that most couples at risk were counseled as to how they could avoid such births. For the policy to be effective, the couples would then have to act to avoid such births.

The question is whether a compulsory screening program would be more effective than a voluntary one. Little reason exists to think that it would be. Although counseling does have some effect in decreasing the number of children couples have, depending on the severity of the disease anywhere from 35 to 75 percent have the same number they planned to have before counselling.[5] Since most of these people were voluntarily counseled, it is unlikely the success rate would be as high among people screened involuntarily. If no significant reduction in births of defective children is achieved, there will be little or no financial savings either. Because of this, and because a mandatory program is an infringement of people's freedom, compulsory screening is not acceptable. Nonetheless, a voluntary program is supportable. Such a program is likely to be more effective because participants will be motivated to avoid the birth of children with defects (the primary reason for coming), and it will increase their freedom to control their reproductive activity.

One might ask at what age such screening should be offered. Many of the mandatory carrier programs screened newborn children. However, the main purpose of carrier screening is to provide information for reproductive decisions—decisions that newborn children do not confront. In a voluntary program, there is no reason for age restrictions. Voluntary programs should, however, be aimed at people before their reproductive attitudes are set. This means that, at the least, general education about genetics and reproduction should begin in elementary school. Actual screening and information about contraception and parenting should occur before reproductive years—in junior high school.

[5]"Genetic Diagnosis and Counseling," *Encyclopedia of Bioethics* (1978), 2, 563.

Prenatal Diagnosis

Prenatal diagnosis includes a variety of techniques designed to provide information about whether a fetus has a defect. The following techniques are currently used. (1) Maternal blood serum can be tested. Such tests for alpha-fetoprotein can determine whether the fetus is likely to have neural tube defects (those in the spine or brain). (2) Ultrasound can be used to picture the fetus. (3) Fetoscopy, which involves inserting a needle-like instrument into the womb, enables physicians to visualize the fetus. (4) Amniocentesis, the most frequent type of prenatal diagnosis, involves using a needle to withdraw some of the amniotic fluid in the womb; the fluid can then be used for a variety of tests. Fetal cells in the fluid are often cultured and the chromosomes examined for defects. Amniocentesis is not usually performed until the fourteenth to sixteenth week of pregnancy, and culturing fetal cells then takes several weeks. Amniocentesis enables tests to be performed to discover most chromosomal anomalies, the most common being Down syndrome, as well as an increasing number of rare metabolic errors. One can also use amniocentesis with fetoscopy to obtain samples of fetal blood to test for sickle-cell anemia and other blood disorders.

So far as is known, all of these techniques are reasonably safe when performed by experienced physicians. At first, there was much concern about the safety of amniocentesis, but subsequent study has shown that the primary risk is inducing a spontaneous abortion in about 0.5 to 1.0 percent of the cases. The type of amniocentesis which involves drawing samples of fetal blood from the placenta has a somewhat higher risk of spontaneous abortion than drawing amniotic fluid. Ethically, these spontaneous abortions differ even from abortions for medical indications; there is no desire or intent to cause fetal death or knowledge that the fetus will die. Ultrasound, a relatively new technique, has been shown to be safe at the levels used, although it is so new that no information exists about its possible long-term effects. Safety is not currently a major issue in prenatal diagnosis.

People undergo prenatal diagnosis for basically the same reasons as carrier screening—to relieve anxiety about defects of the fetus, and to avoid the birth of a significantly handicapped child. In 95 percent or more of the instances of amniocentesis, the fetus is discovered not to have the defect in question. If a defect is found, then avoiding the birth of a child involves a second trimester abortion, around twenty weeks' gestation.

Much of the concern and ethical argument about prenatal diagnosis has centered around the abortion issue, which is discussed in the next chapter. It should be noted, however, that prenatal diagnosis decreases rather than increases the number of abortions.[6] Some women at risk would have an abortion rather than continue the pregnancy. Prenatal diagnosis usually shows that no defect is present, so these women are able to continue the pregnancy without fear of the specific defect. Other women have an abortion because the fetus is discovered to have a defect. However, as the number of those who would have had an abortion but are reassured is greater than the number who have an abortion, prenatal diagnosis decreases

---

[6]See Aubrey Milunsky, ed., *Genetic Disorders and the Fetus* (New York: Plenum Press, 1979), Chapters 5–7.

the number of abortions. Also, some women at risk of having children with defects will become pregnant only if amniocentesis is available.

Case 2.4 Paula is in her late twenties and her husband Quincy is a year or two older. Paula is pregnant for the first time and goes to the genetics clinic to request prenatal diagnosis for Down syndrome, a chromosomal abnormality causing mental retardation. She works in an institution for mentally retarded persons and is anxious about having a child with Down syndrome. The general incidence of Down syndrome is low for someone Paula's age, less than one-half of one percent, although it increases rapidly for women over thirty-five years old and is about two percent for women over forty. Nor is there a history of the condition in her family. Consequently, the genetics clinic denies her request because there is no medical indication for prenatal diagnosis. After a normal pregnancy, Paula delivers a child with Down syndrome.

Ethical Analysis

This case raises the issue of access to prenatal diagnosis. The primary medical indications for it are advanced maternal age (where the risk of a number of chromosomal anomalies is higher), previous spontaneous abortion or birth of a child with a defect, family history of defects, or carrier screening indicating that there is a higher than normal risk of a child with a defect. Should prenatal diagnosis be denied to women who, like Paula, want it even though there is no medical indication? The arguments for offering the service in these cases are that the normal risk of a defect is about one in two hundred, so there is always some risk of a defective fetus. If no defect is found, anxiety is relieved. In Paula's case, because she works with retarded persons, the anxiety was probably greater than for many other women without medical indications.

The arguments against offering prenatal diagnosis in such cases are these: First, a small risk of spontaneous abortion exists and that risk is not worth taking unless there is an above average risk of defect. However, should the genetics unit make this decision about risk, or should Paula? Paula bears the consequences—either a defective child or the loss of a normal one if a spontaneous abortion occurs. The difference between the risk of a defect in her case and the so-called risk cases is certainly less than two percent. That does not seem like a great enough difference simply to take the decision out of Paula's hands.

Second, there are considerations of cost. If Paula is paying, it is her decision to spend her money on the screening. Cost considerations primarily apply if the government is paying for the procedure. The government might conclude that performing the tests on someone in Paula's situation is not cost-effective; that is, the costs of the test will be greater than money saved by not having to provide for defective children whose birth would be averted. One might reply that many other medical procedures do not save money, and the costs of Paula's anxiety and worry as well as the suffering of any defective children should also be taken into account. Nevertheless, given finite resources, the government might reasonably decide not to fund prenatal diagnosis unless patients are in a class for which it is cost-effective; it simply cannot afford to provide all possible medical tests for everyone who wants them.

A third reason against offering Paula the test is a shortage of resources. This point concerns a lack of facilities, usually laboratories, to perform the tests. If there is a shortage, then tests should be reserved for the high risk patients most apt to benefit by avoiding the birth of a defective child. This concern has been a real one in Canada, where some centers have had to consider raising the maternal age indication from thirty-five to thirty-seven because of lack of facilities for providing tests for all women thirty-five years of age or more who requested them. Even so, if there is laboratory room and Paula is not depriving anyone else of access, this reason has no force.

Another reason has been offered for denying prenatal diagnosis even for women at risk. The suggestion is that if adequate treatment exists for the condition, then prenatal diagnosis should not be offered. An example would be galactosemia. The objection to providing the test for this condition is basically the objection against the use of abortion for this reason. Its soundness therefore depends on the ethics of abortion. If abortion at this stage is not prima facie morally wrong, then the principle of burdens to others supports a decision to abort an affected infant. Even if abortion is a prima facie wrong, consideration of burdens to others might outweigh its wrongness. Consequently, prenatal diagnosis can be denied due to the availability of treatment only if abortion for the proffered reason is ethically wrong. As we shall see in Chapter 3, abortion for such reasons is not ethically wrong, so there is no basis for denying prenatal diagnosis.

Another issue that arises in prenatal diagnosis is withholding information. One example has already been broached earlier, namely, withholding the sex of the fetus to prevent a woman aborting for sex preselection. However, other reasons also arise. For example, whenever a chromosomal analysis is performed from amniocentesis, most other major chromosomal anomalies are discovered. Thus, the fetus might be found to have XYY chromosomes. Some evidence indicates that males with an extra Y chromosome (which determines male sex) are more likely to be violent and to become inmates of prisons or institutions for the insane. However, the vast majority of XYY men are not violent or insane, and the evidence of greater risk is uncertain. If parents are told of this characteristic, it might adversely alter the way they raise the child if they decide to continue the pregnancy. Yet the purpose of prenatal diagnosis is to discover information; this is why the woman wants the diagnosis. To withhold information seems contrary to the very purpose of prenatal diagnosis.

As in carrier screening, these difficulties can be clarified by advance agreement. Before prenatal diagnosis is performed, a woman can be advised that all sorts of information might be gained, that the significance of some of it is ambiguous, and that she can have all information gained or only selected parts. In short, it can be agreed in advance what type of information will be imparted. It is up to the woman to decide what information is worth having and what is not. Even if it would be ethically wrong for her to have an abortion for sex preselection or an XYY condition, that is a matter for ethical and policy conditions for abortion, not for information from prenatal diagnosis. Not all women want the information in order to decide about abortion; some of them are simply curious about the sex of the fetus.

Another aspect of agreements prior to prenatal diagnosis should be considered. When prenatal diagnosis began, a number of centers refused to provide it unless the woman agreed to have an abortion should a defect be found. Otherwise, it was claimed, the risks were not worth taking. Today, major centers do not have that requirement. For one reason, the risks of amniocentesis are simply not that great. For another, more than 95 percent of the time no defect is found, and anxiety is relieved; this relief would be denied to women who would not agree in advance to an abortion. Also, the abortion decision, it is claimed, is one which a woman should make without pressure or requirements set by others. Nonetheless, a few private doctors or hospitals may still require such an agreement.[7] For the reasons given, that practice is not ethically acceptable.

These last two issues point out a fallacy in much thinking about prenatal diagnosis, namely, that its sole purpose is to discover fetuses with defects or diseases so that they can be aborted. Probably most medical practices still operate on that assumption, but it is not correct. First, some people may want to be better prepared to care for a child should it be damaged. Major psychological, economic, and living adjustments may be necessary. Second, sometimes steps can be taken to ameliorate the child's condition (see Chapter 6). For example, cesarean section delivery might be advisable to reduce chances of birth injury to particularly susceptible fetuses. Intrauterine treatment is also possible for some defects or diseases. So even people opposed to abortion have reasons for prenatal diagnosis.

Another ethical issue that pertains to carrier screening as well as prenatal diagnosis concerns whether counseling should be directive or nondirective. The pure idea of nondirective counseling is that a counselor provides people with information and assists them in thinking through their decisions, but does not advise, recommend, or influence decisions. In directive counseling, by contrast, a counselor does recommend courses of action to clients.

Nondirective counseling is generally accepted as the ethically appropriate model. The primary reason for this view is to preserve clients' freedom to control their lives. Directive counseling is likely to impose the counselor's or society's values on the client. It logically need not do so; a counselor could always frame recommendations solely in terms of a client's values, but in practice that would rarely occur. Few counselors are trained to recognize or analyze the cultural views of others.

The ideal of nondirective counseling is ethically inappropriate. People want and should be free to make important decisions affecting their lives on the basis of their values. Nonetheless, clients are not always the only people involved. If a pregnancy occurs and proceeds to term, then an affected child is also involved. The principle regarding risk to the unborn provides one reason not to leave decisions completely up to clients.

But the fundamental flaws in the nondirective ideal of genetic counseling are that it is unattainable and ignores features of a model appropriate for

[7]Joe Rubin, "Malpractice Board Urged by MD/Lawyer," *The Medical Post,* December 1, 1981, p. 17.

other medical situations[8] (perhaps because reproductive decisions are considered more a matter of lifestyle than medicine). It is not the mere making of recommendations that deprives clients of freedom, and one can do so without making recommendations. For instance, one can withhold information; nondirective counselors do not always—or perhaps even usually—present all the available options. Nondirective counseling influences clients in a nonexplicit way to conform to the counselor's bias. The tone of voice, body movements, and the language in which information is given can strongly influence clients. Since these aspects are not brought into the open, clients are not likely to recognize their influence. Of course, directive counseling can take a strong, authoritarian, and dogmatic position which also deprives clients of freedom of choice, but then clients can clearly recognize the counselor's intention.

In other medical situations, clients usually ask physicians for recommendations and advice. Clients often ask nondirective counselors for recommendations or what they would do. Many counselors try to avoid answering, thus depriving clients of one of the chief benefits they seek. In short, clients often want more than information; they also want advice and recommendations based on a counselor's experience with the outcomes of other patients. To offer such advice openly in a nonthreatening and explicit manner does not deprive clients of freedom to accept or reject such advice or recommendations. Clients frequently ignore or act contrary to medical advice. However, counselors should make clear that they will assist and support clients whatever they decide, or else they should withdraw from the case.

Policy Analysis

Few policy issues of prenatal diagnosis need to be examined. For the most part, the policies that govern medical practice also adequately deal with prenatal diagnosis, including malpractice based on negligent performance of tests and failure to obtain informed consent. Actual practice in this area may be more deficient (due to failure to offer all options) than in other areas of medicine, but this merely indicates a deficiency in the enforcement of the policies, not in the policies themselves. However, a few specific questions deserve some consideration.

One such issue concerns civil suits by parents against physicians or counselors who have not provided specific information or informed them of the availability of tests. Failure to inform women of the availability of tests when they have medical indications for prenatal diagnosis constitutes negligence, even if such failure is still common practice. Whether failure to provide information constitutes negligence is more complex; it is unclear what information is to be provided, and consent documents do not spell it out.

If parents incur extra expense when a defective child is born due to such negligence, then they should be compensated as in other cases of negligence. The usual legal standard for damages is that plaintiffs should receive compensation to place them in the position they would have been in

---

[8]See Michael D. Bayles, *Professional Ethics* (Belmont, Calif.: Wadsworth Publishing Company, 1981), pp. 69–70.

but for the negligent conduct of the defendant. Thus, one might argue that women or couples in such cases should receive the entire costs of raising the child, because had they been informed, they would have had an abortion and the child would not have been born. (In Canada, abortions are legal only for the physical or mental health of the woman, not merely because of possible defect of the fetus, but in practice, abortion is available in these cases.) However, damage awards might plausibly be restricted to the extra expenses over and above those of a normal child, because the woman or couple was willing and expected to incur those expenses. Moreover, in prenatal diagnosis, one can contend that after aborting an affected child the woman would probably proceed to become pregnant again to have a normal child. In short, had she been adequately informed, it is likely she would have eventually had a normal child. Consequently, the difference between the position she would have been in and the one she actually is in, is that between the costs of a normal and of an affected child.

A more complicated situation arises if an affected child sues a physician, clinic, laboratory, or its parents for damages in what is called a "wrongful life" case. The child claims that it should be compensated for the suffering and extra costs incurred as a result of the negligence. Until a few years ago, children lost all such cases.[9] The central argument used in those cases was that one cannot compare the life of a child with defects to a state of nonexistence, which is the condition that would have prevailed had an abortion been performed or had the child not been conceived. However, that argument is unsound.[10] One can consider the value of that life and compare it to nonexistence, which has a zero value. The child will, however, only be worse off and have suffered damages should its life be worse than nonexistence. Consequently, the child would be entitled only to damages that would bring its life to the level of nonexistence, and to punitive damages if the defendant was grossly negligent. With this basis for compensation, few children would qualify for damages, and the damages to which they would be entitled are probably so slight as not to make it worth suing.

In 1980, a California appellate court did hold that a child born with Tay-Sachs could sue a laboratory that negligently screened its parents for carrier status.[11] As to damages, the court claimed that the inability to calculate damages does not bar recovery for wrongdoing. The child, the court held, was entitled to damages as if it had been injured after conception, but based on its actual life expectancy (four years) rather than that of a normal person (seventy-plus years).

However, this solution has a logical difficulty. Had the parents been informed of their carrier status, this child would not have been born. They would have had amniocentesis and aborted this child. Consequently, it is not possible to square the damages granted with traditional standards.

[9]See, for example, Gleitman v. Cosgrove, 49 N.J. 22, 227 A.2d 689 (1967); Gildiner v. Thomas Jefferson Univ. Hosp., 451 F. Supp. 692 (E.D. Pa. 1978); Becker v. Schwartz, 46 N.Y.2d 401, 386 N.E.2d 807 (1978).

[10]Michael D. Bayles, "Harm to the Unconceived," *Philosophy and Public Affairs*, 5, no. 3 (1976), 295; Clifton Perry, "Wrongful Life and the Comparison of Harms," *Westminster Institute Review*, 1, no. 4 (1982), 7–9.

[11]Curlender v. Bio-Science Laboratories, 106 Cal. App. 3d 811, 165 Cal. Rptr. 477 (1980).

In a subsequent case the California Supreme Court held that a child could not recover for pain and suffering or other general damages, because that would have to be offset by the incidental benefit the child received, namely, life.[12] Juries do not have adequate experience to make such judgments. However, the court held that a child could recover special damages for medical expense, special training, and so forth. The court rested its argument on the traditional standard for damages, but essentially deleted considerations of the value of life versus nonexistence. We indicated above that such evaluations are technically possible, but that they would not usually contribute much in damages. Consequently, the court's omission of this factor is acceptable for legal purposes.

A final policy consideration concerns funding. Most genetic screening and counseling is at least partially funded by governments. In Canada, with its national health insurance system, carrier screening, prenatal diagnosis, and legal abortions are funded. In the United States, prenatal diagnosis is not often covered by government programs such as Medicaid, or by private insurance. Private insurance companies might find it financially beneficial to include prenatal diagnosis for some women at risk because the tests might be less expensive than the cost of medical care for children born with defects. This depends, in part, on how many births of defective children are avoided and how much of the cost of care for defective children the companies would pay. Even were it not financially beneficial, the cost of adding such coverage would often be willingly borne by subscribers.

In Medicaid, of course, the government has refused to fund abortions except to save the life of a woman and occasionally in cases of rape. (This policy is considered in the next chapter.) Given that the government is funding carrier screening for Tay-Sachs, sickle cell, and thalassemia, it is anomalous not to fund prenatal diagnosis and elective abortion under Medicaid.[13] A generally accepted purpose of carrier screening is to enable couples to avoid the conception or birth of infants with defects, and for these diseases this can be accomplished by prenatal diagnosis and elective abortion. The government has simply made this widely accepted approach less available to the poor, implicitly encouraging them instead to avoid conception, use artificial insemination or some other technique, or give birth to defective children who will be cared for at government expense. This policy is acceptable only if abortion of defective fetuses should be prohibited.

BIBLIOGRAPHY

BERGSMA, DANIEL; LAPPE, MARC; ROBLIN, RICHARD O.; and GUSTAFSON, JAMES M., eds. *Ethical, Social and Legal Dimensions of Screening for Human Genetic Disease.* Birth Defects: Original Article Series; The National Foundation March of Dimes, vol. X, no. 6. New York: Symposia Specialists, Stratton Intercontinental Medical Book Corporation, 1974.

[12]Turpin v. Sortini, 31 Cal. 3d 220, 182 Cal. Rptr. 337, 643 P.2d 954 (1982).

[13]See John C. Fletcher, "The Morality and Ethics of Prenatal Diagnosis," in *Genetic Disorders and the Fetus,* ed. Aubrey Milunsky (New York: Plenum Press, 1979), p. 633.

FLETCHER, JOHN C. "Ethical Issues in Genetic Screening and Antenatal Diagnosis," *Clinical Obstetrics and Gynecology*, 24, no. 4 (1981), 1151–68.

"Genetic Diagnosis and Counseling," *Encyclopedia of Bioethics* (1978), 2, 555–66.

"Genetic Screening," *Encyclopedia of Bioethics* (1978), 2, 567–72.

HOLMES, HELEN B.; HOSKINS, BETTY B.; and GROSS, MICHAEL, eds. *The Custom-Made Child? Women-Centered Perspectives*. Clifton, N. J.: The Humana Press, Inc., 1981.

MILUNSKY, AUBREY; and ANNAS, GEROGE J., eds. *Genetics and the Law II*. New York: Plenum Press, 1980.

POWLEDGE, TABITHA M.; and FLETCHER, JOHN "Guidelines for the Ethical, Social and Legal Issues in Prenatal Diagnosis," *New England Journal of Medicine,* 300, no. 4 (Jan. 25, 1979), 168–72.

"Prenatal Diagnosis," *Encyclopedia of Bioethics* (1978), 3, 1332–46.

REILLY, PHILIP *Genetics, Law, and Social Policy*. Cambridge: Harvard University Press, 1977.

RESEARCH GROUP, INSTITUTE OF SOCIETY, ETHICS AND THE LIFE SCIENCES "Ethical and Social Issues in Screening for Genetic Disease," *New England Journal of Medicine,* 286, no. 21 (May 25, 1972), 1129–32.

WILLIAMSON, NANCY E. "Boys or Girls? Parents' Preferences and Sex Control," *Population Bulletin,* 33, no. 1 (January 1978), 3–35.

CHAPTER 3

Abortion

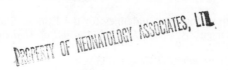

Case 3.1   Rachel and her husband, Sam, are devastated by the news that Rachel is carrying a fetus with Down syndrome. If she carries it to term, they face raising a mentally retarded child. Rachel, who is thirty-seven, followed her physician's advice and had amniocentesis performed. He recommends it for all his pregnant patients over thirty-five years of age. "There's probably nothing to worry about," he said, "but I think you should have the test just to be safe." Rachel had agreed, not really believing it could happen to her.

Rachel has a good job as assistant manager in a large department store. When she and Sam married nine years ago, she insisted that she continue working. While her career went well, she began to want children and she realized she had little time left to have them. Three years ago she had a girl, Tina. She had taken leave from her job to have Tina, but a couple of months after Tina's birth she went back to work. She and Sam then decided that it would be nice to have another child, preferably a boy.

Now their hopes are dashed. If she goes ahead with the pregnancy, she might have to give up her job—possibly forever. A retarded child would need special care and stimulation to develop its full potential. Moreover, the time she might have to devote to this baby might seriously detract from the time she would have for Tina. While she and Sam could probably get along financially, it would be difficult with only his income. Moreover, they might find it hard to adjust to having a retarded child. Some people do so well, but others find it difficult. It might depend on the degree of retardation, but that cannot be accurately predicted at this point. Yet, at her age it is highly unlikely that she can have another child, and the fetus is a boy. She would like to have a loving child. Nonetheless, everything considered, she decides to have an abortion. She has to have it soon; according to the doctor she is already twenty-one weeks pregnant.

Rachel's situation raises one of the most controversial issues in North America—the ethics and legality of abortion. In both the United States and Canada, people vigorously dispute the morality of abortion. In the United States, offices of Planned Parenthood have been attacked because they assist women in obtaining abortions. Lobbying continues for a constitutional amendment which would overturn the Supreme Court decision that women have a constitutional right to abortion before the fetus becomes viable (around 24 weeks of pregnancy). In Canada, legal abortions must be approved by a committee of physicians on the ground that abortion is necessary for the woman's health. The result has been battles between pro-choice and anti-abortion groups for control of the hospital boards which determine whether, and how many, abortions a hospital will perform.

The central question in the abortion dispute is whether it is wrong to kill a fetus, and if it is, what exceptions there are. Abortion can be defined as the termination of a pregnancy prior to normal delivery. The usual medical definition defines it as prior to viability, but that definition implies that abortions cannot occur during the third trimester of pregnancy. For purposes of ethical evaluation, the issue of late-term abortions should be left open. One can argue that abortion need not by definition involve the death or killing of a fetus,[1] for the fetus might be kept alive after removal from the womb. However, with present abortion techniques and medical technology, that is not generally possible during the first two trimesters. Abortion at least involves the foreseeable death of the fetus. If it did not, most of the present controversy would disappear. In this chapter, 'fetus' is used to refer to all stages of development from conception to termination of pregnancy by abortion or birth.

Although the central issue in abortion concerns when, if ever, it is permissible to bring about the death of the fetus, many of the arguments are concerned with rights. Rights are emphasized because the most prevalent reason given for abortion being wrong is that it violates the fetus's right to life. Some people challenge the claim that fetuses have a right to life. Thus, three aspects of abortion must be considered: (1) the moral status of the fetus, (2) ethical implications of that status, and (3) legal policy toward abortion.

A large number of views exist on abortion, but they generally fall into three groups, usually called the conservative, moderate, and liberal views. The main claims of a conservative view are that fetuses have the same rights as other human beings, including the right not to be killed; that abortion is ethically wrong except to save the life of a pregnant woman; and that except to save the life of a pregnant woman abortion should be illegal. A liberal view takes almost an opposite approach to each conservative claim: fetuses are not the sort of beings that can have rights; abortion therefore cannot violate any rights of a fetus and is usually ethically permissible; and abortion on request should be legal. Moderate views cover the broad range in between. Generally, with moderate views, fetuses have some moral status prior to viability; abortions are ethical only at certain times or for specified reasons; and there should be some legal restrictions on abortion.

---

[1]L. W. Sumner, *Abortion and Moral Theory* (Princeton, N.J.: Princeton University Press, 1981), pp. 6–8.

Conservative Views

There is not just one conservative view, but a number of closely related views that give practically the same results. The foundation of every conservative view is the right to life of fetuses.

Status of Fetuses

Most conservatives contend that, from the moment of conception, fetuses have a right to life. A few believe that a right to life does not exist until implantation, about two weeks after conception. The central question is why conservatives believe fetuses have a right to life. A number of reasons have been offered for this claim.

"Human fetuses are human beings. As members of the human species, they have all the rights of other members." In one sense, liberals do not deny that fetuses are human beings—they belong to the human species, not the canine or feline species. This is a factual matter of biological classification from which it does not follow that fetuses have a right to life. The question at issue is whether all members of the human species have moral status, especially a right to life. This conservative contention merely asserts or assumes an answer to it.

"From the moment of conception, a single, living, human entity with a genetic identity exists. Prior to conception, there is not one entity with a complete genetic makeup." Some conservatives use this argument to support implantation as the time fetuses acquire a right to life; prior to that time an embryo can split (identical twins), so identity is not established until then. (This view permits abortifacients such as a morning-after pill.) However, identity alone is not sufficient to establish a moral right to life. Suppose scientists develop the ability to unite particular sperm and eggs in the laboratory. In that case, before a particular sperm and egg were united, the precise genetic identity of the resulting entity would be known, but rational persons would not then think it wrong to fail to unite the sperm and egg, or contend that they had a right to life. Moreover, although genetic identity is established at fertilization (except for the possibility of twinning), until about two weeks the cells are not interdependent and can develop separately.[2] There is not one organism. Thus genetic identity is not sufficient to have a right to life.

"Fetuses have the potentiality in the normal course of events to develop into adult human beings clearly having a right to life. Normal adult human beings have some set of characteristics in virtue of which they have a right to life. Fetuses are potentially such beings; with natural growth and development they will become adult human beings. Therefore, they too have a right to life." The difficulty with this contention is that it uses a potentiality principle: Although X does not have characteristics C, it has them potentially; so it should be treated as though it does. But it is simply a mistake to treat something that is potentially a C as though it is one already. To do so implies that X does not have to be C to be so treated; rather, some

---

[2]Clifford Grobstein, "The Moral Uses of 'Spare' Embryos," *The Hastings Center Report*, 12, no. 3 (June 1982), 6.

other set of characteristics, C', is sufficient. Consequently, one must show that the characteristics a fetus actually has are sufficient for a right to life.

There does not appear to be any other area in which such a principle is used. Fermenting grape juice is potentially wine, but it is not yet wine and it would be a mistake to treat it as though it were. A fourteen-year-old person is potentially a licensed driver and voter, but that does not mean the person now has rights to be licensed to drive and to vote. If one tries to refine the potentiality principle so that it does not apply to these other cases, it is likely to beg the question. Suppose one said that a human entity who presently lacks a right, but in the normal course of events will develop into one who does have that right, should be treated as having that right now. This principle still applies to the fourteen-year-old would-be voter. If one further narrows the principle by restricting it to the right to life, then one essentially repeats what one is to prove: namely, that fetuses have a right to life. Furthermore, the potentiality principle might deny severely defective fetuses and newborn infants a right to life, because in the normal course of events they would not develop into normal adult humans clearly having a right to life.

The potentiality principle appears plausible because we do often treat things in special ways in virtue of what they can become. For example, we take care of pregnant cows and their fetuses so that we can have healthy calves. These cases depend on wanting X to be C. If one does not want X to be C, then one does not accord it the special treatment. In the abortion context, a woman desiring an abortion does not want the fetus to develop into a child. Other people may want the fetus to develop into a child, but that does not imply the fetus has a right to develop into a child. Moreover, most people who want the fetus to develop into a child do so because they think it has a right to life, but that merely begs the question.

"Human fetuses are members of a species the normal adult members of which have a right to life." This contention resembles the claim that fetuses are human beings, and is designed to avoid the objection that the potentiality claim might exclude severely defective fetuses and infants. Human beings normally develop into beings having a right to life in virtue of some set of characteristics. Human fetuses belong to that species, so they have the basic human right to life.

This argument also commits a logical fallacy. It contends that because most members of a class have a set of characteristics, all members of that class should be treated as though they had those characteristics. Obviously, no one would follow that principle in life generally. If the normal apple from a tree develops into a red, juicy, sweet apple, one does not then treat all apples from the tree as though they were red, juicy, and sweet regardless of their actual condition. Such a principle has been the basis of discrimination. Women, perhaps, do not normally have the upper body (shoulder) strength of men, but one cannot thus deny all women jobs requiring considerable upper body strength simply because most of them lack it. One must consider the strength of individual women.

A conservative might reply that this criterion basically asks what rule one would support for beings having a right to life. Good reasons exist to accept a rule giving a right to life to members of the human species. Consequently, human fetuses have a right to life. In short, the right to life extends to fetuses because an acceptable rule ascribes such a right to life to all members of the human species.

The question is whether an acceptable rule might not ascribe a right to life to a smaller group than the entire human species. No reason has been given why such a rule might not ascribe a right to life only to all humans born alive or to some other subgroup. This is especially true if the reasons for a right to life primarily apply to a clear subset of the human species.

Consequently, conservative views are unacceptable. The reasons given to support fetuses's having a right to life all involve logical mistakes. The first simply asserts an answer or begs the question; the second confuses a necessary characteristic with a sufficient one; the third rests on the fallacious potentiality principle; and the fourth treats all members of a class as though they had the characteristics of normal members of that class. Nonetheless, it is important to understand what follows from the mistaken conservative claim about the status of the fetus, because many people misunderstand the conservative views of ethics and policy.

Ethical Claims

Conservative views of the ethics of abortion follow directly from the claim that fetuses have a right to life. If a person has a right to life, it is wrong to kill that person except in certain specific situations such as self-defense. The central question for conservatives concerns when a fetus's alleged right to life might be outweighed by other considerations. Generally, only other rights would outweigh the right to life of a fetus.

Self-defense is a common exception to the right to life. One is entitled to use force and perhaps to kill another person to protect one's life. Thus, if the continuation of a pregnancy threatens a woman's life, she is entitled to have an abortion as a form of self-defense. Most conservatives do allow that abortions are permissible to save the life of a pregnant woman. Some conservatives distinguish between direct and indirect killing of the fetus, permitting only the latter. This issue is not being considered here.

Three aspects of the self-defense rationale need to be considered. First, sometimes it is said that it is wrong to kill an innocent human being. The normal instance of self-defense is when an aggressor attacks a person, and is killed in self-defense. In this type of situation, the aggressor is not morally innocent. Fetuses, however, do not deliberately attack their mothers; they are morally blameless. The concept of innocence employed here is a technical one meaning not seriously threatening another's life. One would be entitled to kill in self-defense were one attacked by a person who was morally blameless due to insanity.

Second, how serious must the threat be? One would not be justified in shooting an attacker who was hitting one with a pillow. In pregnancy, the question is how serious the threat to life must be. A woman with a weak heart faces increased risk of death in pregnancy, but it is far from certain that she will die. No exact criterion is possible here, just as one cannot specify exactly when a threat is serious enough to justify self-defense in other situations. Generally, it must pose a risk significantly greater than in normal pregnancy and childbirth.

Third, must the threat actually be to the woman's life? Generally, people are entitled to kill in self-defense even if they are not likely to die, but only suffer severe physical injury. Thus, some serious threat to physical health might justify an abortion. Conservatives almost always deny that the mental health of a woman will justify an abortion. Perhaps their primary reason is because the mental health criterion is often used to justify almost any abortion. Yet, some threats to mental health plausibly justify killing in self-defense. Suppose another person were about to inject one with a drug that would make one insane for ten years—schizophrenic or manic-depressive. Killing in self-defense in such a situation is surely acceptable. What this person is trying to do will in a sense destroy one's life, as one has known it. Thus, logically, substantial risks of serious mental illness to the pregnant woman would also override a fetus's right to life.

Another right of pregnant women that is often thought to override a fetus's right to life is the right to control one's body. Indeed, this is probably the basic concept underlying the U.S. Supreme Court's decision in Roe v. Wade that women have a right to an abortion, although the court confusingly called it a right to privacy.[3] People generally have a right to control what happens to their bodies, not to be touched unless they consent. This right underlies the law of assault and battery and the requirement of informed consent to medical treatment. If a woman has such a right, then might it not outweigh a fetus's right to life?

At first glance, a right to life seems more important than a right to control one's body. However, one must be more precise about the right to life. Philosophers often distinguish between positive and negative rights. Negative rights are usually characterized as rights that others not interfere. A right to freedom of the press is a right not to have others interfere with publication. Positive rights are usually characterized as rights that others assist in an activity or provide one something. For example, a right to be repaid money loaned is that one be paid the money, not merely that the debtor not interfere in one's collecting it. The right to life has traditionally been considered a negative right not to be killed. Although a fetus is dependent on the woman for nourishment, a right to life does not necessarily include a right to be provided sustenance for nine months. By having an abortion, some people contend, a woman is merely refusing to assist a fetus even though without that assistance the fetus will die. Still, it does not mean that the fetus is entitled to such assistance.[4]

While a right to life does not involve more than a duty of strangers not to kill, in special relationships it often includes a duty of assistance. The parent-child relationship is just such a special relationship; parents have a duty to feed their children. Consequently, a fetus's right to life might well be a positive one with respect to the pregnant woman or someone else in a special relationship.

Such special relationships create positive rights only when they are entered voluntarily; the obligation arises from the special relationship. To

---

[3]410 U.S. 113 (1973).

[4]For a much fuller statement of this type of argument, see Judith Jarvis Thomson, "A Defense of Abortion," in *The Problem of Abortion,* ed. Joel Feinberg (Belmont, Calif.: Wadsworth Publishing Company, Inc., 1973), pp. 121–39.

respect women's rights to their bodies and control of their lives, they cannot be bound if they involuntarily enter the relationships. The principle of freedom of reproduction justified in Chapter 1, that people should not have parental responsibilities involuntarily, is merely a special instance of this more general consideration. If a woman becomes pregnant as a result of rape, she has involuntarily entered into a relationship with a fetus. She thus has no duty to nourish it, despite the fact that the fetus did not intentionally thrust itself upon her.

Some conservatives accept this argument and agree that abortion is permissible in cases of rape. However, they point out, most pregnancies are not clearly involuntary. There are degrees of freedom and voluntariness. Perhaps the closest situation to that of rape is that of a woman who conscientiously practices contraception, but becomes pregnant due to contraceptive failure; even then, she could have completely abstained from sexual intercourse, or been sterilized. If the woman was careless in her contraceptive practice or simply did not practice contraception, then as we saw in Chapter 1, parental responsibility remains. The woman carelessly or knowingly took a chance of becoming pregnant, and that is sufficient to establish her responsibility. Most conservatives hold her responsible for all pregnancies except those due to rape.

Neither of the exceptions to a fetus's right to life—serious threat to the woman's health or involuntary pregnancy—would justify or permit an abortion for Rachel. She deliberately became pregnant, and it is the fetus's mental condition, not her own, that is at stake. It has been suggested that rights of the fetus itself might justify abortions for defective fetuses.[5] No child should be brought into the world unless certain basic requirements are met which make it possible for the child to fulfill future interests. If the child would have no chance for a reasonable life, then it will have been wronged. If a severely defective child is born, it will have certain rights that cannot be fulfilled, and so it will be wronged.

There are difficulties with such an argument. First, it cannot overcome the fetus's right to life unless those rights that cannot be fulfilled are more important than the right to life. Others who accept a similar condition specify that such an argument is acceptable only if the child's life would be so miserable as to justify euthanasia.[6] This would certainly exclude Rachel's situation, because the life of a person with Down syndrome is not so miserable as to justify euthanasia; indeed, most people with Down syndrome are fairly happy. Second, the conduct of parents or others after birth would not violate any rights the child has, because one violates rights only if one fails to fulfill them when one can do so. Moreover, the rights a child would later have are not rights a fetus currently has, so no rights of a fetus would be violated if it were not aborted. At best, this argument would justify abortion for fetuses whose lives would be so miserable that euthanasia would be justifiable. Whether or not euthanasia would ever be justifiable is discussed

[5]See Joel Feinberg, "Is There a Right to Be Born?" in *Understanding Moral Philosophy*, ed. James Rachels (Encino, Calif.: Dickenson Publishing Company, Inc., 1976), pp. 346–57, esp. pp. 356–57. He does not suggest that these rights overcome a right to life, for he denies that fetuses have a right to be born. See also Sumner, *Abortion and Moral Theory*, pp. 156–57.

[6]Sumner, *Abortion and Moral Theory*, p. 156.

in Chapter 5. In any case, the argument will not support a conservative making an exception and permitting abortion in a case like Rachel's.

The principle regarding risk to the unborn (defended in Chapter 2) also fails to support an exception to a right to life. It does avoid the problem of ascribing to a fetus rights that a child would have, because it does not rest on rights at all. However, it was developed for decisions prior to conception, so its justification assumed that no being had a right to life to overcome. Consequently, it cannot override a right to life. However, if, as will be argued later, fetuses do not have moral status and a right to life, it will apply. It will then imply that it is wrong *not* to have an abortion if there is substantial risk that the child will have a significant defect.

Policy Claim

The standard conservative view is that abortion ought to be illegal at any stage of gestation, except to save the life of a pregnant woman. A few conservatives also permit abortion in cases of rape. None of them accepts legal abortion for fetal defects.

Several liberal objections to the conservative claim that abortion should be illegal rest on misunderstandings. Liberals object that conservatives are imposing their religious views on others. In the United States, this violates the ideal of separation of church and state. However, although most Roman Catholics are strongly committed to the conservative view, so are many Orthodox Jews, Protestants, and others. More important, the above presentation of the conservative view makes no reference to any religious doctrine; the conservative view can be argued on a completely secular moral basis and need not impose any religious view.

Some liberals also object that conservatives are simply legislating their own moral views, and that in a democratic society with pluralistic moral views, one ought not legislate private morality. Instead, tolerance should prevail; conservatives can act on their moral views and liberals on theirs. However, conservatives are not appealing to some private secular morality. Their claim is that the law should prohibit violations of the rights of others; abortion violates fetuses' rights to life; it causes harm to them; and the law ought to prohibit conduct causing such harm to others. Conservatives are no more enforcing a private morality than are those who support laws protecting other people from being killed. Liberals who make this criticism simply fail to take seriously the conservative view that fetuses have a right to life like any normal adult human being.

Another objection is that making abortion illegal leads to the death of many pregnant women in bungled illegal abortions, to say nothing of injuries short of death. This liberal objection also fails to take seriously the conservative claim that fetuses have a right to life. Conservatives accord pregnant women as well as fetuses a right to life. But, on the conservative view, every abortion involves the loss of a life. More lives are saved than lost by legally prohibiting abortion. Conservatives are not indifferent to the well-being and lives of pregnant women; they simply take fetal lives equally seriously.

Given the conservatives' mistaken premise that fetuses have a right to life, their basic policy position is unassailable even on liberal legal principles. At best, one can argue that perhaps physical and mental health, rape, and severe fetal defect should be recognized as exceptions, along with that of saving a woman's life. From a policy point of view, conservatives can make a plausible argument for not allowing these other exceptions even if they are ethically sound. Such exceptions can be and have been used by many women to obtain abortions in situations that would not ethically justify overriding a fetus's right to life.

Although the conservative view is consistent, it is unacceptable. The crux of the conservative view is the claim that fetuses have a right to life from conception (or implantation). As shown above, this premise is not acceptable. All the arguments for it involve logical mistakes. Thus, the entire conservative view rests on a mistaken premise. We must look elsewhere for an acceptable view.

Liberal Views

As we have seen, abortions for the mental health of a pregnant woman occur far beyond the scope which conservatives would believe justifiable. The following case is an example of just that sort. In Canada, where the sole legal ground for an abortion is the health of the pregnant woman, cases like it often result in legal abortions. It is also typical of cases liberals believe are justifiable.

Case 3.2 Ursula is a seventeen-year-old high school junior who lives with her mother and younger brother. Her mother and father have recently divorced, and her mother, who has not worked for a long time, is taking a refresher course to brush up her secretarial skills and get a job. Ursula's boyfriend of six months, Victor, has just started college. Ursula consulted her doctor about contraception and tried an oral contraceptive for about half a month, but quit due to spot bleeding and pain.

Ursula is about two months pregnant. Although she has known for ten days that she is pregnant, she did not confide in her mother until now. Both her parents are quite upset. Her mother has always opposed abortion, but is inclined to think that perhaps Ursula should have one; her father strongly favors abortion. He says he cannot afford to support Ursula and her child as well as his ex-wife, his son and himself, and will not help Ursula financially. Nor can Ursula find a job; during the recession jobs are hard to find, especially for pregnant seventeen-year-old high school dropouts. Victor is supportive, but he clearly does not want to marry Ursula, at least at present. Nor does he want to tell his parents that Ursula is pregnant. Although his father has been laid off from the local Ford assembly plant, his parents still give him financial support for college.

Initially, Ursula wants to carry the fetus to term whether or not Victor marries her. However, after a couple of weeks of thinking about it, she decides an abortion would be best for her. If she were to carry the fetus to term, she could not afford to provide for the child. Neither her mother, father, nor Victor could provide much (if any) financial support. Without finishing high school, she is unlikely to find a job that pays well. Moreover, her education would probably be finished, and she thinks it likely Victor would never marry her if she had the baby and did not finish school. In this situation, not only would having a child be disastrous for her life, but she would not be able to provide her child with many opportunities. If she could find a job, she would be unable to stay home and care for it as she would like.

Clearly, Ursula's case is not one in which conservatives would find abortion ethically permissible. Her health is not in such jeopardy as to justify taking the life of the fetus. Nor is she involuntarily pregnant. Although she did not intend to become pregnant, she was careless or reckless in not using contraception. Although the child would lack many advantages were she to carry it to term, no reason exists to think that its life would be worse than nonexistence.

Status of Fetuses

Liberals believe abortions in cases like Ursula's are ethically permissible. Indeed, they generally support abortion on request. The crux of the liberal position is the denial of any moral status for fetuses. If fetuses have no right to life or other serious moral claim, then there is no reason to think abortion is ethically wrong. Liberals deny that fetuses have moral status because they lack those characteristics in virtue of which normal adult humans have a right to life. To have a right to life, one must actually have those characteristics—not have them potentially or be members of a class of beings most of whom have them.

The central problem for liberals is to specify the characteristics by virtue of which beings have a right to life. This has turned out to be a difficult task. One prominent argument for a liberal view is the following.[7] To have a right to life, a being must have the capacities to envisage its future, to desire future states of itself, to have self-consciousness, and to have the concept of a self; it must also be a self and now be or have been self-conscious.[8] Unless a being meets these conditions, one cannot violate its right to life. Violating a right involves in some way frustrating a corresponding desire. Unless beings can desire their own continued existence, they cannot have a right to life, for no desire can exist to be frustrated. A full account of this argument involves many qualifications and conditions to take care of odd cases, but the above conveys the central idea. As fetuses do not have the capacities for self-consciousness and the concepts of a self and its continued existence, they cannot have a right to life.

One objection to this view is that since newborn infants also lack these capacities, they do not have a right to life either. Only some time after birth would human infants acquire a right to life. For practical purposes, a liberal might adopt the principle that newborn infants have a right to life after one

[7]Michael Tooley, "A Defense of Abortion and Infanticide," in *The Problem of Abortion*, ed. Joel Feinberg (Belmont, Calif.: Wadsworth Publishing Company, Inc., 1973), pp. 51–91.

[8]*Ibid.*, pp. 59–60, 89.

week.[9] Although this consequence may seem abhorrent, that does not provide a logical reason for rejecting it. Attitudes and beliefs may have to be revised in light of logic and information.

Perhaps the central difficulty in this argument is the claim that there must be a close connection between desiring something and having a right to it. People can have many rights to things they do not in fact desire, for example, to be professional wrestlers. However, the argument does not assume that one must actually desire something to have a right to it, only that one must be capable of desiring it. But even this claim seems too strong. Mentally ill persons can have rights to property even though they do not now, and perhaps never will, have the capacity to understand their property. Even competent adults can have rights to things and yet lack the capacity to desire them, for example, to make complicated legal arrangements. Thus, in general, there is not the close connection between desiring something and having a right to it that this view assumes.

A similar liberal approach is to pick out a set of characteristics that normal adult humans have that seem to justify ascribing a right to life. For example, people with a right to life "are conscious, have a concept and awareness of themselves, are capable of experiencing emotions, can reason and acquire understanding, can plan ahead, can act on their plans, and can feel pleasure and pain."[10] Any being that has these characteristics surely has a right to life.

The aim is to provide a set of characteristics each of which is necessary and which together are sufficient for a being to have a right to life. The above set is surely sufficient, but is each necessary? A person paralyzed from the neck down is unable to act on many plans, but having all the rest of the characteristics is sufficient for the person to have a right to life. Psychopaths or sociopaths are immune to most emotions, but that does not appear sufficient to deny them a right to life.

There probably is no set of characteristics that are each necessary and jointly sufficient for having a right to life. More likely, some characteristics are necessary, such as the ability to feel pleasure and pain, and at least some of the others must be present. If this is so, fetuses might lack some necessary characteristics. If not, one must consider precisely what characteristics fetuses have at different stages of development to determine whether they have enough to have a right to life.

The liberal view of the moral status of the fetus rests on the correct claim that, to have a right to life, fetuses must actually possess those characteristics which give normal adults that right. Liberals claim that fetuses lack at least one of the characteristics necessary to such a right. The liberal difficulty lies in specifying precisely what characteristics are necessary for normal adult humans to have a right to life. It is easy to provide a set of sufficient conditions; but to deny that fetuses have a right to life, one must specify some necessary trait that is lacked by fetuses.

[9]*Ibid.*, p. 91.

[10]Joel Feinberg, "Abortion," in *Matters of Life and Death: New Introductory Essays in Moral Philosophy*, ed. Tom Regan (New York: Random House, 1980), p. 189. Copyright © 1980 by Random House, Inc.

Since liberals deny fetuses moral status, they are inclined to conclude that abortion is ethical and should be legally permissible on request at any stage of pregnancy. Two particular aspects of liberal views require further consideration.

The first aspect concerns the ethics of abortion. Liberals need not find all abortions ethically permissible; they simply cannot object on the ground that fetal rights are violated. A liberal need not consider an abortion for purposes of mere sexual preference ethically acceptable. Most people would object to such an abortion because the reason is pernicious or at least too trivial. This suggests that having an abortion is wrong unless one has a good reason, and that sex preference is not a good reason. But why is abortion wrong without a good reason? An answer is likely to appeal to the moral status of the fetus, but a liberal cannot give this sort of response.

Nevertheless, a liberal can respond that having an abortion for sex preference indicates a moral defect in the pregnant woman. It indicates an irrational and unethical sexist attitude. Thus, the woman's decision is made on ethically inappropriate grounds. A liberal can make similar arguments about other reasons for abortion, such as not wanting to be pregnant during the heat of the summer. Such a person lacks an appropriate concern for the seriousness of reproductive decisions.

The second aspect of the liberal position concerns the ethical and legal prohibition of infanticide. As noted above, some liberal arguments imply that newborn infants also lack a right to life. If so, then there does not appear to be a basis for prohibiting infanticide. All liberal views are likely to face this problem, because it is difficult to show that newborn infants have any characteristics which viable fetuses lack, and by virtue of which normal adult human beings have a right to life. Still, liberals do not have to permit infanticide on request. Conduct can be ethically wrong or illegal for reasons other than violation of rights. Thus, liberals might contend that permitting infanticide would seriously affect the concern and tenderness that people have for infants, brutalize medical personnel, and so forth. Theoretically, liberals could use such arguments to support ethical or legal proscriptions of abortion, but in fact they almost always use them only to prohibit infanticide.

Conservatives thus ascribe a right to life to fetuses, and then have difficulty supporting abortion even in the most deserving cases. Liberals deny fetuses any moral status, and then have difficulty restricting infanticide. Interestingly, conservatives are apt to favor prohibiting abortions by law even when they might be ethically justified by their own theory, for example, when pregnancy risks severe mental illness. Liberals are likely to favor permitting abortions that are ethically wrong. The reason for this difference between the two is (as discussed in the Introduction) that legal policy and ethics do not rest on the same grounds. That something is ethically permissible does not necessarily imply that it should be legal, and that something is ethically wrong does not necessarily imply that it should be legally prohibited.

Conservatives would claim that abortions for both Rachel (Case 3.1) and Ursula (Case 3.2) are ethically wrong and should be illegal, while liberals would claim that both are ethically permissible and should be legal. Neither view is acceptable. Conservative arguments for fetuses' rights to life are mistaken. Liberal arguments fail to show that fetuses cannot have a right to life. Perhaps a moderate approach between them can provide an acceptable view.

Moderate Views

Status of Fetuses

A large variety of moderate views is possible. One approach has been to ascribe gradually increasing moral status to fetuses as they develop. Such a view, it is claimed, better accords with biological development. The more developed fetuses are—the greater their gestational age—the stronger the reasons needed to justify abortion. Thus, during the early stages of fetal development, say during the first trimester, many reasons will justify an abortion because such fetuses have little moral status. At two months, Ursula's reasons for wanting an abortion would probably justify having one. During the second trimester—say at five months—they probably would not.

This type of moderate view has not been adequately justified by its supporters. The crucial problem is that no characteristic or set of characteristics has been specified to support this developing moral status. The view assumes that reasons are needed to justify abortion at any stage of fetal development. Thus, some moral status is ascribed to the fetus from conception, or at least very early development, but no characteristics have been identified that would justify this status. Various aspects of the fetus develop—human shape, neurological capacity, and so forth—but these features need to be shown to be a basis for ascribing moral status. Moreover, the moral status must vary directly with these characteristics.

At best, this gradualist approach would have to ascribe moral status—a right to life or duty not to have an abortion—at conception and vary its strength over the gestational period. Unfortunately, without picking out the characteristics and explaining why they support such a status, the view is not acceptable. It may be more in accord with many people's attitudes or gut feelings than is the conservative view, but that is not a reason to accept it, for the question is what those attitudes and feelings ought to be. Perhaps one could defend such a view indirectly; that is, without ascribing moral status to fetuses. One could appeal to effects on adults and society, much as liberals support legal prohibitions of infanticide. But the prospects for that appear unlikely; liberals do not find compelling the extension of the reasons from prohibition of infanticide to prohibition of abortion.

Another moderate approach specifies a point in development at which fetuses acquire moral status and a right to life. Instead of gradually acquiring moral status during development, prior to some point the fetus has no moral status, and after the point it has full status. Historically, there have been several such points when fetuses have been thought to acquire moral status: when brain activity begins (at about six weeks),[11] at quickening (when the mother can feel the fetus move), and at viability, for instance. Once the fetus has reached this point, it has a right to life, and the general outlines of the conservative view apply.

Wayne Sumner has provided a strong defense of one such position which also fits with the utilitarian tradition in ethical theory.[12] Sumner contends that the capacity for sensation, for feeling and emotional affect, confers moral status. Good and bad, that which is valuable and harmful in life, concerns psychological states. Thus, the capacity for such states should provide moral status. Although fetuses probably acquire sentience gradually, one can determine that somewhere in the middle of the second trimester, say, during the fifth month, fetuses have a capacity for it.

Sumner fails to distinguish between having some moral status or other and having that particular moral status, namely, a right to life, most important for the abortion debate. He correctly concludes that animals have moral status (not to be tortured) because they have sentience. But he does not show that animals or fetuses should have a right to life. It is plausible to ascribe different rights depending on different characteristics. Moreover, Sumner sets the time at which moral status is acquired so early because he appeals to evidence that the capacity for awareness is present, that is, that the anatomical structure for awareness is present. However, the actual presence of awareness or sentience, not the mere capacity for it, is necessary. Unless sentience is actually present, at least part of the time, no feelings or affect, no good or bad mental states occur. If lives do not have good or bad, then there is no basis for moral status.

Ethical and Policy Claims

Moderate views of the type Sumner defends pick some point in fetal development to ascribe a right to life. Prior to that point, fetuses have no rights and abortion is permissible on the grounds liberals defend. After that point, abortion is permissible only for reasons of the sort conservatives accept. In Sumner's view, after the fifth month of pregnancy abortion is permissible only for the health of the pregnant woman or for a fetal defect that would justify euthanasia in a newborn.[13] This means that Ursula in Case 3.2 can ethically have an abortion, but Rachel in Case 3.1 cannot. The question for Sumner is when in her pregnancy Rachel is to have an abortion. He would not consider an abortion after twenty weeks of gestation, or perhaps a couple of weeks earlier, ethically permissible. Given present techniques of amniocentesis, it is often close to twenty weeks, and sometimes later, that diagnosis of Down syndrome and many other defects can be made and an abortion scheduled. Because Down syndrome does not imply a life

[11]See Baruch Brody, "On the Humanity of the Fetus," in *Abortion: Pro and Con,* ed. Robert L. Perkins (Cambridge, Mass.: Schenkman Publishing Company, 1974), pp. 69–90, for a defense of such a view.

[12]Sumner, *Abortion and Moral Theory,* Chap. 4.

[13]*Ibid.*, p. 156.

worse than nonexistence, late abortion of a fetus affected with it (and many other conditions for which fetuses are often aborted) would not be justified by Sumner's "eugenic" or fetal defect ground. Thus, he gives a result different from either the conservatives (who would not allow an abortion in either case), or the liberals (who would allow abortion in both cases).

Persons holding a gradualist approach are likely to agree with the liberals on the ethics of the two cases. Since Ursula's abortion would be early in the pregnancy, her reasons are strong enough to justify it. Although Rachel's abortion would be later and so would require a stronger reason to justify it ethically, most gradualists believe that a fetus with Down syndrome would provide such a justification. Unfortunately, because the gradualists do not specify the characteristics that give moral status, it is not clear how one determines which reasons are acceptable at various stages of gestation and which are not. Usually, one only has their statements that this or that reason ethically justifies an abortion at some gestational age.

The gradualist moderate approach has considerable difficulty determining an acceptable legal policy. A law simply stating that increasingly strong reasons are needed as the pregnancy progresses would not work well. Consequently, gradualists are apt to favor a complex law like the following: Abortion is permitted on request in the first three months; is permitted only for a number of specified reasons such as the woman's health, a fetal defect, and so on during the second three months; and is permitted for few reasons if at all during the final three months. Such a law is difficult to administer. The more distinctions there are, the more likely the law will be applied unequally. Moreover, more resources are required to administer it, or else it is largely left to the medical profession to follow, with sanctions only for gross violations.

Moderates of the other type support a law that permits abortion on request until the time a fetus has a right to life, and then only for a few specific reasons—the pregnant woman's life (or health) and perhaps serious fetal defect. Such a law is easier to administer than a gradualist law. But, unless the time a fetus acquires a right to life is rather late or the exceptions are broad, there will be considerable pressure to violate it. For example, if, like Sumner, one sets the date at about twenty weeks, there will be considerable pressure to make exceptions for fetal defect.

In general, these moderate views have fewer problems than either conservative or liberal views. The primary flaws concern inadequate explanations of the moral status of the fetus. Thus, if that aspect can be clarified, an acceptable view is likely to emerge.

An Acceptable View

Status of Fetuses

For fetuses to have moral status, they must be capable of good or bad in their lives. What happens to them must make a difference to them. Consequently, some form of awareness is necessary for moral status. As we saw in discussing Sumner's view, fetuses acquire sentience during the fifth month of pregnancy. However, sentience alone does not appear sufficient to ground a right to life. It can provide moral status and rights only with respect to the good and bad that merely sentient beings can experience (pleasure, pain, and primitive emotional states)—rights not to be caused unnecessary suffering.

Evidence indicates that fetuses are conscious around the end of the seventh month of pregnancy. Somewhere between twenty-eight and thirty-two weeks of gestation, the brain's neural connections are as complete and advanced as those of newborns. Moreover, shortly thereafter they have distinct sleeping and awake brain waves.[14] In short, in the third trimester (about the seventh month), fetuses are conscious, can taste, feel, see, hear, learn, and maybe remember at a primitive level. Thus, they can perform about half the activities on the earlier list sufficient for adult human beings to have a right to life. In addition, at this stage, fetuses are viable and can live independent of the pregnant woman. While this does not constitute a conclusive case for ascribing a right to life, fetuses after the seventh month do have a large number of the characteristics that are sufficient to ascribe a right to life to normal adult humans. No conclusive reason can be given that these are sufficient in themselves, but it is not clear that fetuses lack any necessary condition.

Thus, during the seventh month, fetuses do not appear to lack any necessary characteristic for a right to life. This point corresponds roughly with viability, being perhaps a bit later. Viability does not give fetuses moral status, for it changes with medical advances; but the other characteristics fetuses have at that point do. If fetuses were not then viable, they would still have these characteristics and a plausible claim to moral status.

Ethical Analysis

The sentience of fetuses at about the fifth month confers some moral status, but not a right to life. Ethically, it implies that they should not be caused unnecessary suffering. Consequently, from this time any abortion should use the least painful technique. Practically, this implies that saline abortions, which plausibly cause more pain than abortions using prostaglandins, ought not to be used.

As we have seen, plausible reasons exist for holding that at about seven months fetuses have enough characteristics for a right to life. The question is whether good reasons exist for accepting an ethical rule ascribing a right to life to fetuses from seven months on. We can approach this by considering the reasons for accepting a rule prohibiting killing normal adults.[15] Killing causes harm to victims by the fear of being killed, the actual killing, and the loss of valuable life. It brutalizes the killer, who loses respect for the right to life. It causes grief for friends and others who love the

[14]Thomas Verny with John Kelly, *The Secret Life of the Unborn Child* (Toronto: Collins, 1981), p. 41.

[15]See Sissela Bok, "Who Shall Count as a Human Being? A Treacherous Question in the Abortion Discussion," in *Abortion: Pro and Con,* ed. Robert L. Perkins (Cambridge, Mass.: Schenkman Publishing Company, 1974), pp. 98–99.

victim. Other people also have an increased fear of being killed. However, many of these reasons do not apply (or not as strongly) to killing fetuses.[16] Although it may lose a valuable life and suffer in the actual killing, a fetus is not capable of fearing abortion. It is unlikely that abortionists are brutalized like ordinary killers. Many physicians strongly dislike performing abortions, which indicates that they have not become brutally insensitive. The grief of a woman and others for a fetus is usually less than for an adult. Finally, other people do not have reason to fear for their lives.

Some other reasons might apply to fetuses but not adults. The central one is that society has special attitudes toward children—infants and children are treated with special care and tenderness. This attitude is important for the nurturance of children; they must receive special protection and care to grow up to be capable, moral members of society. A callous attitude toward fetuses could threaten this special attitude. Furthermore, many people who would like to have children cannot; it is an especial affront to them for a woman to abort a viable fetus that they could adopt were it delivered alive. As fetuses delivered after seven months could be available for adoption, aborting them causes unnecessary unhappiness.

Consequently, although the direct reasons for a rule against abortions after the seventh month of fetal development are not as strong as for a rule prohibiting killing adults, in terms of harm to the fetus and violation of its rights, sufficient reasons exist to accept such a rule. The fetus at that point has many of the characteristics by virtue of which normal adults have a right to life. And others are willing and able to care for the child after birth.

Consequently, it is rational to ascribe an ethical right to life at about the end of the seventh month of fetal development. Until that point abortions are permissible for any reasons liberals will accept. Not any abortion decision is ethically permissible; decisions to have abortions on grounds of sex preference can be condemned as unethical because of what they indicate about the sexual bias of the pregnant woman. Others can be condemned for similar reasons.

From twenty-eight weeks or so onwards, abortions are ethically justifiable only for the sorts of reasons conservatives might accept (although not all do). Abortions for pregnancy caused by rape or contraceptive failure are not really a problem at this point, because such pregnancies should have been terminated much earlier. Neither is the pregnant woman's health often a practical reason for abortion at this point. Almost always, if a woman's health is in danger, the fetus can be delivered by cesarean section—the same technique (hysterotomy) as is generally used for very late abortions. Nonetheless, should a situation arise in which the woman's health is seriously in jeopardy and the fetus must be killed, such an abortion would be justifiable. Similarly, abortions for fetal defect are unlikely during the seventh month and later. Defects can be detected earlier and abortions performed then. Nonetheless, should a serious defect not be determined until this stage, abortion would be ethically justifiable on the grounds that it is permissible to allow a newborn defective infant to die. Those grounds are discussed in detail in Chapter 5.

[16]*Ibid.*, pp. 99–100.

If a fetus ethically ought not be caused unnecessary suffering from the fifth month on, one might think that the law should specify abortion techniques after that point. But such a law would be difficult to enforce, and medical developments might quickly make such a law out-of-date. Consequently, such judgments can be left to the medical profession unless practice diverges greatly from policy considerations.

Given that fetuses do not acquire an ethical right to life until about the seventh month of pregnancy, unless there are policy considerations to the contrary, abortion should be legally permissible on request until then. No exact date can be set by the arguments given, but the date should be around twenty-eight weeks. The legislature must draw a sharp line so that people can know precisely what is permissible.

One consideration favors an earlier time. With increasing gestational age, more aborted infants will be born alive. The use of prostaglandins rather than saline injection increases the chances of this. Moreover, many are apt to suffer damage such as blindness and mental retardation. To avoid the problems created by such infants, earlier abortions are preferable. However, this cannot be justified by the fetuses' right to life. It would be ethically permissible on that basis to use some painless technique to ensure that a fetus is not born alive, but that might brutalize physicians. It does not appear essential that the law set an early date, but physicians should (as they do) encourage earlier abortions and undertake later ones (after twenty-four weeks) only after considering the risks of the fetus being born alive and the harm it could suffer.

After the point determined by the legislature, abortion should be legally prohibited except for serious threats to the pregnant woman's health when cesarean delivery is not possible, and for quite serious fetal defects. The fetal defect exception would be the same as that for allowing newborns to die. (Such a standard is developed in Chapter 5.) In practice, these exceptions will probably not be very important, because genuine cases for their application are apt to be rare.

A related issue concerns what should be done with infants who are alive after a later permissible abortion. The intent obviously was that the fetus not live. One might argue that such fetuses should be permitted to die whatever their condition because that was the original expectation. The pregnant woman did not plan to have a child. However, mothers cannot simply let their newborn infants die because they do not want them. As the fetus is no longer dependent on the woman, her right to control her body is no longer affected. Moreover, if she does not want to care for the child, she can surrender her rights to the child. Consequently, the law should protect such infants as it should any others born alive. Infants with defects should be treated the same as other defective newborns.

Another policy question is whether the consent of the genetic father should be required for an abortion. Depending on her relationship with the father, a woman ethically should consult him. The question here, however, is whether the law should require the father's consent to an abortion. The U.S. Supreme Court and English courts have held that the father's consent is not necessary.[17] In practice, the requirement of a father's (or parents, for legal minors) consent amounts to a veto over a woman's decision for an abortion. Should the woman not want an abortion, the father could not legally force her to have one. The father's consent would only make a difference if a woman wanted an abortion and the father did not. The father would be able to require the woman to continue the pregnancy by withholding his consent. This would give the father control over the woman's body. He would have such control even when there was no fetal claim sufficient to override the woman's right. In effect, then, it would simply give fathers a right to control women's bodies because they wanted the children. Indeed, were such a right granted, no clear principle exists to distinguish such cases from those in which a male wants an unwilling woman to become pregnant. Consequently, paternal consent should not be required.

Nor should the law require that genetic fathers be informed and consulted. Some genetic fathers do not care. If the relationship between the pregnant woman and genetic father is good, she will probably do so anyway. If it is not, such a requirement is likely to make it worse, or the woman will probably ignore his views. Also, a woman who does not want to inform the genetic father, but continues to have a relationship with him, probably fears informal coercion. Consequently, such a law would probably do little good and might cause much harm.

The last policy question to be considered caused much controversy in the United States during the late 1970s, namely, funding abortions. The issue concerned whether Medicaid insurance must pay for legal abortions for women otherwise qualified for Medicaid health care. Legally, the issue involved some complex questions of interpreting the Social Security Act, which established Medicaid.[18] These questions are ignored here. The central moral issue concerns whether the government ought to pay for legal abortions for those who cannot afford them.

Many people who favor government funding argue that it is incident to a woman's right to an abortion. A right to an abortion they claim, does not have practical value if a woman cannot afford one. Because the government pays for childbirth, if it does not also pay for abortion it in effect supports one option over the other, and infringes the right to an abortion. Those opposed to government funding (mostly conservatives opposed to abortions except to save a woman's life) argue against funding because the money is used for immoral purposes. A right to an abortion, they claim, does not mean a right to have one provided.

Does a woman's right to an abortion imply that the government ought to pay for abortions for women who cannot afford them? This chapter has not argued that women have a right to an abortion. Rather, the argument has been about whether it is wrong to have an abortion. The general conclusion was that during the first seven months of pregnancy, fetuses have no moral status establishing a right to life, so abortions should not be legally prohibited. That is, abortions are permissible. At best, to say that conduct is permissible is to establish a sort of negative right; in particular, a right that

---

[17]Planned Parenthood of Central Missouri v. Danforth, 428 U.S. 52 (1976); Paton v. British Pregnancy Advisory Service Trustees, [1978] 3 W.L.R. 687 (Q.B.D.).

[18]See Harris v. McRae, 100 S.CT. 2671 (1980).

the law not interfere by prohibiting an abortion. Such a right gives no basis for assistance in having one.

Perhaps the rights that underlie acceptable exceptions to a prohibition of abortion would establish a right to have abortions funded. The right to control one's body supports abortions only in cases of rape or other involuntary pregnancies. A right to health, which underlies the self-defense justification and is in the Medicaid law, would apply only to abortions when a woman's health was threatened. The fetal defect exception does not rest on any right of the woman, except as her health would be affected. These rights would at best support a claim to funded abortions in cases of rape or threat to the woman's health.

The so-called Hyde Amendment to appropriation bills, which prohibits U.S. federal Medicaid payments for most abortions, has varied in different years but has never allowed payment in all these situations. Cases of rape have sometimes been allowed and sometimes not. Sometimes payment has been allowed only for abortions necessary to save the life of the woman. Payments have never been allowed for abortions for a woman's mental health. Supporters of the Hyde Amendment argue that if mental health were included, then in practice all abortions would be funded. In Canada, cases like Ursula's are granted on mental health grounds, so their argument is likely correct. Here one faces the problem that the law cannot practically enforce the finer distinctions that ethics can make. In any case, even if payment were made for abortions for all the reasons supported by rights, it would not cover cases like Ursula's or even Rachel's, unless their mental health was likely to be affected by having the children.

Although the rights of women in abortion do not support government payment for abortions except in cases of rape or threat to health, it does not follow that there are not good reasons for government funding of abortions. A large number of reasons can be offered—overcoming poverty, population control, the possible harm to unwanted children, and financial savings to government. These reasons cannot be developed here; they lead beyond the scope of this book.

Even if such reasons are found persuasive for government funding, conservatives have a final objection to it. They perceive most abortions as seriously wrong. They are conscientiously opposed to abortions except to save the life of the pregnant woman; perhaps to prevent serious threat to her health; and perhaps in cases of rape or incest. To preserve their moral integrity, they do not want to participate in any way in what they consider grossly immoral activity.

This claim deserves respect. People should not be forced to act contrary to their informed moral beliefs, even if those beliefs are incorrect. Conscientious objectors are permitted during war, when the very existence of government is at stake. However, even then the conscientious objection extends only to active participation in the war effort, not to withholding taxes.

Even allowing conservatives' conscientious objection to participating in the funding of abortion through their taxes need not prevent government funding of abortions. A variety of schemes can be used to permit conservatives not to contribute to abortions. They could be permitted a tax credit for the amount of their contribution to abortions not necessary for health reasons. Or, as with presidential election campaigns, a check-off system could be used for those who want to help pay for abortions. If half the taxpayers in the United States were to check off a contribution of about $2.00 to fund abortions not necessary to save a woman's life, a fund could be established that would be adequate to fund all such abortions for women on Medicaid. Conservatives might still object to any government participation in funding such abortions, but at this point their objection is very weak. Such funding requires a complex organization, it is most efficiently administered through a program already paying for other health care, and the reasons advanced—poverty, financial savings, and so on—are appropriate governmental purposes.

Despite the presence of universal government-funded health care, this precise issue has not been prominent in Canada. The reason is simply that abortions are legal in Canada only on grounds of the pregnant woman's health. Thus, in principle, the government does not pay for abortions to which conservatives object. In practice, as has been pointed out, abortions for cases like Ursula's and Rachel's are available. Provinces differ as to whether they will pay for abortions obtained in the United States which might be illegal in Canada. But in Canada the practical controversy has focused on whether hospitals will offer abortions and if so, how many. The right to an abortion for one's health is clearly a negative right. It is an exception to a criminal law prohibiting abortions; such an exception cannot be interpreted as a positive right. Because hospitals are thus free to set up abortion committees and perform legal abortions or not, the controversy has focused on such committees and on numerical quotas for abortions, not on funding.

Abortion in the 1970s was a source of much social debate and conflict, and this dispute continues into the 1980s. It continues because it concerns very fundamental ethical principles—the right to life and the prohibition of killing. Moreover, it arises on the borderline of the moral community; it concerns who will be counted as members of that community. A variety of positions is available on the issues, but they boil down to three basic types: conservative, liberal, and moderate.

This chapter has argued for a moderate position toward the liberal end of the spectrum. Most abortions prior to somewhere around twenty-eight weeks are ethically permissible, except when the reasons indicate a moral defect, such as sexual bias, in the person deciding. After about the twentieth week, a fetus should not be caused unnecessary suffering. From about seven months of pregnancy, a fetus has a right to life. From that time, abortions are ethically permissible only for rape, substantial threat to a pregnant woman's health, or serious fetal defect, and are rarely necessary. The law should permit abortion on request until about twenty-eight weeks of pregnancy, and after that only for maternal health and fetal defect. The woman's rights which underlie permitting abortions do not support government funding of them except for reasons of rape and maternal health. However, other reasons exist for government funding of abortions, especially for poor women. Conservative arguments that they should not be forced to pay for abortions contrary to their consciences are not a bar to government funding.

BIBLIOGRAPHY

CALLAHAN, DANIEL *Abortion: Law, Choice and Morality.* New York: The Macmillan Company, 1970.

FEINBERG, JOEL "Abortion," in *Matters of Life and Death: New Introductory Essays in Moral Philosophy,* ed. Tom Regan. New York: Random House, 1980.

———— "Is There a Right to be Born?" in *Understanding Moral Philosophy,* ed. James Rachels. Encino, Calif.: Dickenson Publishing Company, Inc., 1976.

————, ed. *The Problem of Abortion.* Belmont, Calif.: Wadsworth Publishing Company, Inc., 1973.

Harris v. McRae, 100 S.CT. 2671 (1980).

NOONAN, JOHN T., JR. *A Private Choice: Abortion in America in the Seventies.* New York: The Free Press, A Division of Macmillan Publishing Co., Inc., 1979.

————, ed. *The Morality of Abortion: Legal and Historical Perspectives.* Cambridge, Mass.: Harvard University Press, 1970.

PERKINS, ROBERT L., ed. *Abortion: Pro and Con.* Cambridge, Mass.: Schenkman Publishing Company, 1974.

Roe v. Wade, 410 U.S. 113 (1973).

SUMNER, L. W. *Abortion and Moral Theory.* Princeton, N.J.: Princeton University Press, 1981.

CHAPTER 4

Childbirth

don't copy this page

The focal point of reproduction is the birth of a healthy, normal baby. In the past, concern with the result has led to neglect of the process of birth. North American culture is product-oriented rather than process-oriented; it is whether you win or lose that counts, and all that counts. The process is valued only for its ability to produce a good product. In reproduction, this has meant that the dominant attention has been on mortality and morbidity outcomes of the infant and mother.

In the 1970s, a reaction developed to this product-oriented thinking about childbirth. The reaction has a connection with the women's movement, for women have been subjected to various degrading and insensitive treatments by male-dominated obstetrics. It is also part of a widespread consumer movement.

Whatever its origins and causes, this movement challenges childbirth practices which were accepted almost without question during the 1950s and 1960s. The challenges have gone to almost all aspects of previous childbirth practices: the supine position for delivery; the use of anesthesia, drugs for inducing labor, and electronic fetal monitoring; cesarean section delivery; delivery by physicians rather than midwives; and use of hospitals for delivery. The challenges have sometimes been quite radical, vitriolic, and unreasonable. The defense by the medical establishment has often been reactionary, vicious, and unreasonable. In short, the debate has stirred deep emotions on both sides.

Before considering the issues, it is useful to present some models of alternative approaches to childbirth. There are three parameters of each model: where childbirth occurs, who assists, and how it is done. Underlying these parameters are two theoretical aspects: how childbirth is conceptualized, and the relative emphasis on the safety and quality of the birthing experience. The four models sketched below are ideal types. Many variations and combinations are possible and actually used.

The standard hospital. This model has been and probably still is the dominant one, although elements of it are changing. Childbirth occurs in a hospital obstetrics unit. A physician attends the birth along with a team of nurses. All modern technology is used, as the physician sees fit. The woman labors in a special room, lying on a bed, often attached to an electronic fetal monitor, with a nurse checking occasionally to see how the labor is progressing. When the infant is about to be delivered, the woman is moved to the delivery room where she is given a drug for pain, an IV is started, a small incision is made to widen the birth channel (episiotomy), and anesthesia may be administered. When the baby is born, it is whisked off to the nursery and the doctor is congratulated for his work. In anywhere from 5 to 25 percent of the cases, because of fetal distress or other concerns, the woman is totally anesthetized and the baby delivered by a cesarean section operation.

Childbirth is conceptualized, perhaps unconsciously, as pathological; or if not pathological, certainly as a very dangerous physiological process, and as something the physician does, while the woman's role is passive. It is treated as an illness. The physical safety of mother and infant is the dominant consideration, and the quality of the personal experience secondary.

Hospital birthing center.[1] Childbirth occurs in a hospital, but the setting is quite different from that of the standard hospital model. Rooms are homelike, with regular beds (perhaps queen-sized), dressers, comfortable arm chairs, and other decorations. The birth may be attended by a nurse-midwife or a physician. Technology is used much less, and pain-killing drugs are used sparingly. Electronic fetal monitors are rarely used and the woman is generally free to walk around and visit with her family until time for delivery. The woman's mate or other friend assists in natural childbirth. (We shall use 'natural childbirth' to mean vaginal delivery by a conscious woman with few or no drugs, that is, little or no technology being used.) Immediately after delivery the mother may hold the baby, which stays in a crib in the room (rooming-in). If all goes well, both mother and baby will be released in one or two days.

Women are screened for the likelihood of complications before they are allowed to give birth in the unit, so childbirth is conceptualized as a normal physiologic process that may have dangerous complications requiring removal to a standard obstetrical setting. The pregnant woman is more active, and the attendants have a lesser role. Because the process is considered usually to be safe, more attention is devoted to the quality of the experience for the woman and her family than in the standard hospital.

Birthing center.[2] A birthing center is quite similar to a hospital birthing center, but it is located in another building, sometimes a large house,

[1]For an account of one such center, see John J. Barton and others. "Alternative Birthing Center: Experience in a Teaching Obstetric Service," *Am. J. Ob. Gyn.,* 137, no. 3 (1980), 377–84.

[2]For descriptions of this type of setting, see Byllye Y. Avery and Judith M. Levy, "Contrasts in the Birthing Place: Hospital and Birth Center," in *Birth Control and Controlling Birth: Women-Centered Perspectives,* ed. Helen B. Holmes, Betty B. Hoskins, and Michael Gross (Clifton, N.J.: The Humana Press Inc., 1980), pp. 231–38; and Ruth Watson Lubic, "The Impact of Technology on Health Care—the Childbearing Center: A Case for Technology's Appropriate Use," *J. Nurse-Midwifery,* 24, no. 1 (1979), 8–10.

often close to a hospital. In addition to homelike rooms, a birthing center may have a kitchen where snacks or meals can be prepared. The chief attendant is usually a nurse-midwife, sometimes a physician. Little technology is used, and the woman can usually deliver in whatever position is most comfortable for her, such as squatting. Again, the newborn infant will stay in the room and perhaps the woman's mate will sleep with her. Both woman and child can leave for home about twelve hours after birth.

Childbirth is conceptualized as a normal physiologic process not likely to have dangerous complications, in part because patients at significant risk have been screened out. The birthing center concept perhaps assumes the process is less dangerous than the hospital birth center does, and the pregnant woman may have a somewhat greater role. The quality of personal experience is emphasized even more. However, various medical facilities are available for resuscitation and other care, and difficult cases are transferred to a backup hospital.

Homebirth. When childbirth occurs at home, the chief attendant is likely to be a nurse or lay midwife, although it might be a physician. The attendant brings some equipment, but does not use drugs, forceps, or other technology unless it is considered essential. If the attendant is not a physician, a physician is usually on call if needed; the woman is taken to a hospital in case of significant complications. Many "complications" such as breech presentation might be handled at home.

Again, women are screened in advance for risks, and birth is considered a normal physiologic process that rarely involves danger. The woman is the primary actor in the birth. The quality of the personal experience is heavily emphasized, because safety is not considered a pressing concern, although preparation is normally made for the possibility of a dangerous situation.

Case 4.1 Wilma and Xavier live in a small community in the West. He is a petroleum engineer, and she has a college degree in English. They have decided that they will have only one child, and they are both ecstatic when Wilma becomes pregnant. Wilma has already decided that she wants a natural childbirth. There are only three doctors in town who deliver babies. She is already a patient of Dr. Yale, the only one who, according to her friends, actually encourages and supports natural childbirth. Although the other two say they do, several of her friends who have gone to them told her that at the last minute the doctors had decided the pain was too great. They had then anesthetized them, and delivered the infants in the standard hospital fashion.

In the first few months of her pregnancy, Wilma reads a lot about childbirth, she reads about other women's experiences with homebirths, and gradually develops a conviction to have her baby at home. This is the only one she intends to have, and she and Xavier want it to be a very special occasion that they can remember the rest of their lives. Besides, the local hospital does not have rooming-in or a birthing center. On her next visit, when she is four-months pregnant, Wilma tells Dr. Yale that she wants to have the baby at home and asks him to deliver it there. She explains why she has come to that conclusion. However, Dr. Yale asks her how she can possibly think of risking her baby's health and life by having a homebirth. "It's too dangerous," he says. "Complications can always arise even though a woman like you appears to be developing normally." Wilma replies that of course she does not want to take any big chances. If anything indicates that she will not have a normal delivery, she will go to the hospital; but she has read statistics indicating that for low-risk mothers there is no more danger in delivery at home than at a hospital. Indeed, she says, she has read a book by a doctor who says, "Your own bedroom is safer than the hospital delivery room, and the hospital nursery is infinitely more threatening to your baby than a crib next to your bed."[3]

However, Dr. Yale refuses to deliver her baby at home. He is perfectly willing to go along with any reasonable thing she wants to make the birth as rewarding as possible for her, but the risks are simply too great not to deliver in the hospital. The American College of Obstetricians and Gynecologists, he notes, has declared that the hazards of labor and delivery "require standards of safety which are provided in the hospital setting and cannot be matched in the home situation."[4] Consequently, he says, if she persists in the idea of having the baby at home, he will cease giving her prenatal care.

As Wilma leaves the doctor's office, she is furious. She would do nothing to jeopardize her child's or her own health. But she has read that about half of the births in Holland are at home, and Holland has lower infant mortality rates than the United States. "Besides," she thinks, "it's my baby and my decision as to where I have it. What business does Dr. Yale or the medical profession have telling me where I must or must not have it?"

Value Analysis

In this case, Wilma and her physician appeal to a number of desires or values in childbirth. To arrive at a reasonable judgment about the ethics of various childbirth practices, we must first sort out the rationality of the various desires or values involved. Much of the disagreement between Wilma and Dr. Yale stems from a different weighing of these values, although there is also much disagreement about factual matters involved in the childbirth controversy.

Physical health. Both Wilma and Dr. Yale desire the life and physical health of herself and the baby. Little argument is needed to establish the rationality of a desire for physical health, because health is a precondition for engaging in many activities.

---

[3]Robert S. Mendelsohn, *Male Practice: How Doctors Manipulate Women* (Chicago: Contemporary Books, Inc., 1981), p. 141.

[4]Quoted in Richard H. Subry, "The American College of Obstetricians & Gynecologists: Standards for Safe Childbearing," in *21st Century Obstetrics Now! Vol. 1*, ed. Lee Stewart and David Stewart (Chapel Hill, N.C.: NAPSAC, Inc., 1977), p. 20.

Psychological experience of woman and infant. Women generally want childbirth to be a rewarding personal experience. Fear, drugs that dull mental alertness, and lack of personal attention are among factors that decrease the value of the experience for them. One study found that among a variety of factors of care during pregnancy and delivery, women were least satisfied that doctors understood their feelings and explained the medications administered.[5] Although the majority of women were satisfied with doctors in these respects, a higher percentage was satisfied with the hospital staff's handling of these matters.

A second desire is for attachment or bonding with the newborn infant. The practices of immediately taking an infant away from a mother to the nursery and of putting drops in the infant's eyes decrease the opportunity for such bonding. A major study by two physicians found these aspects quite disruptive of the maternal-infant bonding.[6] As bonding significantly improves the mother's relationship with and affection for the child, this is an important value.

Social. Wilma also wants to share her birthing experience with Xavier. It is their child, not simply hers. Recognizing the importance of shared experiences with loved ones for a life found worthwhile, they want to share the experience as much as possible.

Wilma did not raise the point, but another consideration is the cost of various types of childbirth. In the United States, a standard hospital delivery can cost over $3,000, while other forms are considerably less expensive. The shorter time spent in a birthing center reduces expenses. Moreover, much of the expense of childbirth is paid for through private or public insurance systems. It is rational to reduce the expenses of childbirth as much as possible, consistent with realizing other values. Physicians, of course, desire to maintain or increase their incomes, but this desire might conflict with a similar desire on the part of nurse-midwives, and with the desires of patients and society to keep costs down.

Physician comfort. Although rarely discussed, a significant factor in physicians' decisions is avoidance of personal discomfort. Sometimes this consideration is made explicit; for example, two physicians discussing the value of nurse-midwives in their practice noted a significant decrease in "the aggravation factor"—patient phone calls disrupting their sleep.[7] Many persons charge that various elements of obstetrical practice, including the supine position and the induction of labor, are primarily for the physician's comfort. However, in the childbirth situation, a physician's rational desire for comfort is not as important as the other values involved. Indeed, the other values should take precedence, and physician comfort should be con-

[5]Harriet K. Light, John Senzek Solheim, and G. Wilson Hunter, "Satisfaction with Medical Care During Pregnancy and Delivery," *Am. J. Ob. Gyn.*, 125, no. 6 (1976), 827–31.

[6]Marshall H. Klaus and John H. Kennell, *Maternal-Infant Bonding: The Impact of Early Separation or Loss on Family Development* (St. Louis: C. V. Mosby Company, 1976), esp. 94–96.

[7]T. Schley Gatewood and Richard B. Stewart, "Obstetricians and Nurse-Midwives: The Team Approach in Private Practice," *Am. J. Ob. Gyn.*, 123, no. 1 (1975), 36–37.

sidered only when the other factors are fulfilled as far as reasonable. After all, physicians are being paid for their work and discomfort.

Ethical Analysis

Decision Making

In Case 4.1, Wilma's final question—What business does the medical profession have telling me where and how I must or should deliver my baby?—is a central one concerning childbirth. Who should decide about the aspects of childbirth? Two "decision maker" principles are relevant to answering this question and other forms of the "Who should decide?" question. (1) A good reason for a person to decide a matter is that the person has relevant special expertise. (2) A good reason for a person to decide a matter is that the person will bear the consequences of the decision. The expertise principle is acceptable, because persons with expertise are more likely to make correct decisions than are other persons. By definition, expertise implies a knowledge others do not have, and knowledge simply means that one is correct about certain matters. It is also appropriate to take into account who will bear the consequences, because people who bear consequences are more likely to take the decision seriously than those who do not. Moreover, people rationally desire to control their own lives and decide what happens to them.

Applying these principles to childbirth decisions is rather complex. It is often claimed that physicians have expertise about childbirth, so they should make the decisions. But physicians' expertise primarily concerns the safety of childbirth. Even here, some critics claim that physicians do not have nearly as much knowledge and expertise as they claim, or at least do not act on it. These critics contend that many practices of standard hospital delivery, such as the supine position, the use of drugs and anesthesia, fetal monitors, and cesarean section deliveries, are hazardous to the health of the mother and infant and are often used when their benefits do not outweigh their hazards. To the extent that physicians disagree about the appropriate use of these techniques, or that studies provide conflicting evidence, physicians lack expertise. One cannot have knowledge justifying decision making when evidence is contradictory or uncertain.

More significantly, physicians do not necessarily have expertise relevant to the other values involved in childbirth—the psychological and social factors. They do have expertise concerning their own comfort, but that value is the least important one in the childbirth situation. Moreover, it introduces a conflict of interest between physician comfort and the physical, psychological, and social values of parents. Consequently, the claim of physician expertise is largely limited to considerations of physical safety which are well-documented and accepted on the basis of scientific evidence.

On the other hand, it is claimed that the woman bears the consequences. She is the one giving birth, so she should make the decisions. While this claim is largely correct, one important factor limits this consideration: the baby. Since after seven months gestation the fetus has moral status and a right to life, effects on it must be considered. In short, the fetus will bear consequences as much as or more than the mother. The principle concerning risk to the unborn thus applies to childbirth as much as to conception and abortion. Consideration of the fetus can limit the woman's claim to make decisions, because the fetus also bears the consequences.

The fetus cannot make decisions for itself; someone must decide on its behalf. The question then is who best represents the interests of the fetus—the mother, the physician, the medical profession, or society? Many physicians claim that they best represent the interests of the fetus. They do not deny that almost all women are interested in the well-being of their baby, but the woman's interests can conflict with those of the baby. For example, the woman's interests in the psychological and social aspects of birth are probably greater than those of the child, and women might sacrifice the physical safety of the fetus for their own psychological fulfillment. Even if maternal-infant bonding is beneficial for the baby, it is not as important as its physical well-being. Moreover, it is precisely in the area of physical safety that physicians have expertise. Consequently, it is claimed, they should make the decisions about childbirth.

In opposition to this argument, one can claim that physicians are perhaps so committed to the physical well-being of the infant that they risk the physical health of the mother. Although the causal connection is controversial, the use of electronic fetal monitors has coincided with a significant increase in the rate of delivery by cesarean section. In some hospitals, cesarean deliveries have increased four- or five-fold. Cesarean deliveries pose a greater risk to maternal health than vaginal deliveries, and it is not clear that the increased health of the infants outweighs the increased ill health of mothers. Uncontested data as to the effect of increases in cesarean delivery on infant health do not exist, so one cannot make a comparison with the corresponding risk to maternal health.

This whole medical approach makes two assumptions. First, it tries to make the best of the worst possible outcome, no matter what the likelihood of its occurring.[8] Insufficient thought is given to lesser harms that might be wrought in trying to decrease the risk of the worst outcome. Second, it considers only physical safety in judging outcomes. Other values are not considered. Moreover, the emphasis is on the safety of the fetus. One physician has aptly summarized this whole approach: "Every child has a right to be born safely—every child. It is not justifiable to play the averages, to take chances, to play the odds with the life of a fetus."[9]

Neither assumption is acceptable. Physical health does not always outweigh other considerations. Psychological and social values can outweigh risks to physical health. It might be objected that while one can risk one's own physical health for other values, it is never justifiable to risk the health of others. But this claim is too strong. Parents can reasonably increase the risk of physical injury to their children by purchasing less safe but less expensive automobiles. One must compare the values at stake.

[8]See Howard Brody and James R. Thompson, "The Maximin Strategy in Modern Obstetrics," *J. Fam. Prac.,* 12, no. 6 (1981), 977–86.

[9]Phillip L. Badia, "Medical Ethics Case Conference," *Medical Humanities Report,* Medical Humanities Program, Michigan State University (Winter 1982), 3.

Moreover, the strategy of always minimizing chances of poor physical outcome (worst-case strategy) cannot be justified. There does not appear to be any way to justify one attitude toward risk rather than another. Consequently, physicians cannot argue that their strategy is rationally required or that a strategy of maximizing the average or usual outcome is irrational. There is something grossly incongruous about a strategy of maximal physical safety in the first few minutes or days of life. When the baby leaves the hospital, this attitude is not ethically required; if it were, most children would spend the first years of their lives in a padded room protected from physical injury and infection.

Given conflicting evidence about the safety of delivery of "low risk" pregnancies, and given the possibility that psychological and social factors justify some risk to physical health, women should make the primary decisions about childbirth, within certain limits to protect the interests of the fetus. The primary principle for these limits is that concerning risk to the unborn, which prohibits taking substantial risks of significant damage or defect. What this principle concretely implies is debatable. The strongest clash comes between the homebirth and standard hospital models of childbirth. Consequently, by considering homebirth and limits to it, the overall limits can be fairly well established. If homebirth is acceptable with certain conditions, then the other models of childbirth are too. Of course, birthing centers might be acceptable even if homebirths were not.

Assessing Risks

The two central questions about homebirth pertain to the absence of high technologies for use in case of complications, and the qualifications of birth attendants. The absence of various technologies for handling complications indicates that high-risk deliveries ought not to occur at home. The serious risks are to the infant, not the mother. Even with homebirths involving complications, mothers have a very small chance of dying. Rather, it is the infant whose life and health are most at risk. The principle regarding risk to the unborn implies that it would be wrong for a woman to take a high risk of infant injury and death for psychological benefits primarily for herself.

The difficult questions concern what constitutes high risk, and what percentage of pregnancies is apt to be in that category. Over 90 percent of births could occur with vaginal delivery and no significant injury. The percentage is lower in many hospitals because physicians are quick to do cesarean deliveries. But the percentage with normal outcomes does not indicate the percentage at significant risk of problems. Determining the high-risk population involves indicators of high risk. Among possible indicators are twins, breech presentation, and women with heart problems, diabetes, or low incomes (probably related to poor nutrition, prenatal care, and so on). Each of these conditions has been handled satisfactorily in nonhospital situations, but the chances are poorer. In any case, certainly fewer than 50 percent of women fall within any realistic definition of high risk.

Even if only low-risk women deliver at home, some percentage will develop complications requiring transfer to a standard hospital situation. What percentage this will be largely depends on the criteria for initial selection, the equipment available at the home delivery, and the attitude and skills of the attendant. Statistical evidence can be misleading. Often, data on out-of-hospital births include unplanned deliveries by women not screened for low risk.[10] In any event, perhaps around 25 percent of deliveries pose sufficient risk that, taking into account the danger to the infant, it is unjustifiable for a woman to deliver outside of a hospital. Many of these cases might be delivered in a hospital birthing center. This percentage is only a rough estimate; it could be greater or smaller depending on individual attitudes toward, and empirical beliefs about, risks.

One might object to this conclusion that since even low-risk women can have complications, one cannot apply statistical data to individuals. Any low-risk pregnancy could develop complications. If delivered at home, some of these cases will result in injury to the mother or child. However, this objection rests on the worst-case strategy. It merely points out that some preventable injuries will occur. But that is the risk taken. One can also note that some preventable injuries will be avoided, namely, those resulting from inappropriate medical interventions such as the use of forceps. What the objector wants, but cannot ever get, is the certainty that no preventable injury or harm will occur.

The second central question about homebirths concerns who should be the attendant. An official of the American College of Obstetricians and Gynecologists has claimed that in the United States one should conform to the standards of the World Health Organization, which exclude untrained or uncertified midwives.[11] The difficulty concerns precisely what these standards mean. Apparently everyone now agrees that certified nurse-midwives are competent to handle normal deliveries provided they have medical backup. So the question basically concerns lay midwives. No rational woman would want to be attended by a completely untrained person, such as myself. Lay midwives, however, usually gain experience and knowledge by working with other midwives, although some have simply gotten started accidentally, by being the only person available for a birth. Although most states are abandoning the practice, some still allow lay midwives to be certified. As a minimum, it is wrong to plan a birth without having a trained attendant. Certification by the government is simply one method to ensure that persons have the requisite competence. From an ethical perspective, one could be assured of competence without such certification. Whether that should be permitted as a matter of policy is another matter.

To sum up, homebirth is ethically wrong if the delivery is a high-risk one, or if there is no competent attendant. Precisely what constitutes a high-risk pregnancy is disputable, but on any reasonable standard no more than one-half of pregnancies should be so classified, and homebirth is probably ethically wrong in a much lower percentage of cases than that; even 25 percent seems generous. Nurse-midwives are now generally recognized in the United States and many other countries as capable of handling normal births without the presence of a physician. Consequently, it is ethically permissible for at least one-half of births to be planned, at-home, low-risk deliveries assisted by nurse-midwives.

[10]Warren H. Pearse, "Editorial: Home Birth," *JAMA*, 241, no. 10 (1979), 1039.

[11]*Ibid.*

The Ideal Childbirth

So far, we have considered only what would be ethically wrong. A different question is what the ethically ideal childbirth is. Obviously, the ideal involves a vaginal delivery with a healthy mother and infant. Whether that be by natural childbirth or with drugs, fetal monitors, and anesthesia is more debatable. Given the general safety of the delivery, the other factors are psychological and social ones that can best be judged by the women themselves, with the exception, perhaps, of the economic costs to society. Not all women will judge the same; what is best for one woman will not necessarily be so for another. Some women are more averse to pain than others, and so want pain-killing drugs; others take the safety of their babies as paramount. Consequently, the ethical ideal is a childbirth that takes adequate precautions for the safety of women and babies and permits women to determine for themselves the other aspects of the childbirth experience.

During much of this century, North American women have had little control of their birthing experience. The medical profession has claimed that only physicians are capable of making the decisions. The attitude of the medical profession toward what constitutes a good childbirth has altered significantly during the past decade, so that family-centered childbirth is now considered the norm.[12] Physicians' attitudes that the decisions are theirs to make have not changed nearly as much. Yet, for women, having control over the birthing experience, and deciding for themselves between real alternatives, contributes much to childbirth as a psychologically rewarding experience. Until women have a real choice between homebirths, birthing centers, hospital centers, and standard hospital birthing, the ethical ideal cannot be achieved for most women. Given such choices, the majority of women are perhaps likely to choose a hospital birthing center. But whatever they in fact choose, the central ethical principle is that the choice belongs to women, not to individual physicians, the medical profession, or society.

This fundamental ethical principle extends to how the birth takes place with respect to the use of drugs, anesthesia, electronic fetal monitoring, position, use of intravenous fluids, episiotomies, and all the other elements. Physicians should provide unbiased factual information about the various alternatives and techniques and make recommendations on all these matters. Women should seek such information so that they can make informed choices. Within the limits of the principle regarding risk to the unborn, the decisions should be those of pregnant women.

Physician Refusal

In this context, we can consider the ethics of Dr. Yale's refusal in Case 4.1 to continue to provide Wilma with prenatal care if she plans on a homebirth. First, provided she is not a high-risk case, Wilma's choice to have the birth at home is ethically permissible if she has a competent atten-

---

[12]See Interprofessional Task Force on Health Care of Women and Children, *Joint Position Statement on the Development of Family-Centered Maternity/Newborn Care in Hospitals* (Chicago, Ill.: American College of Obstetrics and Gynecology, 1978).

dant. The only way Wilma can know whether her pregnancy is low risk is to have continued prenatal care. Ethically, she must also have a competent attendant. If she cannot obtain both of those conditions, she cannot ethically have a homebirth.

However, physicians should be free to determine, within certain limits set by society, the conditions under which they will practice. It would greatly restrict physicians' freedom to have to provide whatever services patients desired. So limiting physicians' freedom of choice is no more acceptable than it would be for other persons. Nonetheless, Dr. Yale was in the business of providing prenatal care along with childbirth attendance. His reason for refusing to continue prenatal care was solely to force Wilma to decide as he thought she should. It was a clear instance of coercion by withdrawing care he had already agreed to provide, although he had also expected to provide certain further care.

The central difficulty in the case is that alternative care of the sort Wilma wants is not available. Under those conditions, Dr. Yale's withdrawal of services forces Wilma to choose between an unethical course of conduct (inadequate prenatal care) or complying with his desires for hospital delivery. The question is whether in such circumstances a physician is ethically wrong to withdraw services. The doctor is wrong to withdraw the prenatal care. So far, Wilma has not decided on an unethical course of action. In asking Dr. Yale to continue his prenatal care, she is not asking him to do something he does not normally do or that he believes is unethical. Moreover, he has a professional obligation to continue care until an alternative can be found.

If all goes well and at the time for the delivery Wilma has been unable to secure a competent attendant, Dr. Yale faces another choice. Either he abandons Wilma to an unethical course of conduct (homebirth without a competent attendant), or he provides home delivery. The doctor cannot soundly claim that it would be unethical to provide home delivery if Wilma's is a low-risk case. For as we have seen, with his care it would not be unethical. His grounds for refusing would have to be that because of peer pressure, comfort, income, and so forth he limits his practice to hospital deliveries. Yet, if Wilma persists and has her baby at home without a competent attendant, the physician has not done anything ethically wrong, for the decision then is Wilma's. It is within the discretion of a physician to limit practice to hospital births or to provide attendance at homebirths.

The underlying problem in Wilma's case is the absence of alternative services. This does not necessarily result from unethical conduct by particular persons, but from a structural feature of the provision of health care. The underlying problem is one of policy, not personal ethics.

Policy Analysis

A number of policy issues pertain to childbirth. Most of them are not matters of legal policy but of policies of organizations such as professional medical groups or hospitals.

A semi-legal issue concerns whether homebirth amounts to child abuse. A physician and one-time official of the American College of Obstetricians and Gynecologists once claimed that it does.[13] Such a blanket claim is incorrect. As we have seen, homebirths for low-risk pregnancies with competent attendants are not unethical, and so not child abuse. Some homebirths could constitute legal child abuse; to do so they would have to involve a clearly dangerous pregnancy or not have a competent attendant. The vast majority of planned homebirths do not fall into such a category.

Case 4.2 When Zenia's labor pains begin early one morning, her husband Ambrose takes her to the hospital. Zenia has already had twins, but she is upset by this pregnancy. During the pregnancy, she had two operations for gallbladder disease. Due to her weight problem (she weighs about 350 lbs.), the doctors did not even recognize that she was pregnant. Now they judge her to be healthy except for her obesity. She is attached to a fetal monitor.

About noon a physician tells her that the fetal monitor and other evidence indicate that her fetus is in distress. The physician recommends that they perform a cesarean section delivery, but Zenia refuses. Later a psychiatrist examines her and finds her competent. Ambrose and Zenia's parents ask her to reconsider the cesarean delivery, but she continues to refuse another operation.

At five o'clock, a judge and lawyers come into her room and hold a hearing. The hospital's lawyers ask the judge to order Zenia to have the operation. She has a lawyer to represent her views and another lawyer represents her baby. The judge declares that the baby is a neglected child and orders a cesarean operation to safeguard its life. Zenia then reluctantly complies. The baby is born quite healthy.[14]

This case raises the issue of child abuse or neglect even in the hospital setting. To what extent should a pregnant woman be permitted to ignore medical advice for the well-being of her fetus? In this case, the cesarean operation promised decreased risks for the fetus but somewhat increased risks for the woman. Essentially, the question is one of weighing these risks. There is no evidence that Zenia was especially concerned about psychological or social values; she appears to have been concerned primarily about the risks of the surgery. The main value at stake is that of safety, and the woman may be biased toward her own well-being. Physicians are experts on risks to physical safety and their avoidance. Thus, the decision-maker principle of expertise seems to indicate that physicians should decide.

However, before we so conclude, we must recognize that we are now considering legal policy, not merely ethical matters. The court deprived Zenia of freedom to control her body. She was legally compelled to undergo an operation, albeit not a very dangerous one. One would not generally accept the state's right to compel one person to undergo medical treatment

---

[13]Warren Pearse, *Obstetric-Gynecology News,* 12, no. 1. (1977), 33; quoted in Helen Swallow, "Midwives in Many Settings," in *Birth Control and Controlling Birth: Women-Centered Perspectives,* ed. Helen B. Holmes, Betty B. Hoskins, and Michael Gross (Clifton, N.J.: The Humana Press Inc., 1980), p. 248.

[14]See Watson A. Bowes, Jr., and Brad Selgestad, "Fetal Versus Maternal Rights: Medical and Legal Perspectives," *Ob. Gyn.,* 58, no. 2 (1981), 209–14. The names in the text were invented for stylistic reasons.

for the benefit of another. Yet, this case differs, because Zenia is the mother and parents have a duty to care for their children. Had Zenia failed to risk her life to save her two-year-old child who was drowning in a swimming pool, she would properly have been held legally liable. Consequently, it is acceptable for courts to require pregnant women to undergo medical treatment and some risks for their unborn children.

Nonetheless, the courts should require stringent proof of the risk to the child. In Zenia's case the child was born healthy. Two commentators remark that this "simply underscores the limitations of continuous fetal heart monitoring as a means of predicting neonatal outcome."[15] In short, physicians got a judge to order surgery on the basis of weak evidence of fetal distress. Some such results must be expected when statistical evidence is used, but it is questionable whether external fetal monitors, especially on an obese woman, should justify a legally compelled operation.

Yet a further condition must apply. The likely benefits to the fetus must substantially outweigh the risks to the woman. Her right to control her body is being overridden. A slight benefit is not enough to do so. Thus, a court should have clear and convincing proof that the risks of harm to the fetus would constitute child neglect or abuse after birth should the woman fail to act in ways risking her health to a similar degree as the treatment.

The principle involved here can apply prior to childbirth.[16] For example, a court might intervene to detoxify an alcoholic woman or a drug addict. Both conditions risk significant harm to an unborn child, and the woman's interests in consuming alcohol or drugs are certainly less weighty than those of health. Besides, in these cases, but not others, the woman will also benefit. One might think that this principle would not apply prior to seven months gestation when the fetus has developed sufficiently to have a right to life. However, this is not true. The point, as with the principle concerning risk to the unborn of which it is a policy application, is to avoid harm to a child born alive. Thus, a woman could be held to have such a duty until she aborts or has firmly decided to abort.

Another policy question concerns whether a physician would be guilty of professional misconduct simply by attending a homebirth. The Alberta (Canada) College of Physicians and Surgeons has declared that, except in emergencies, a physician would be.[17] Again, this claim is based on an inadequately supported belief that homebirths are too dangerous. It is another instance of the worst-case strategy. A general rule that it is professional misconduct for a physician simply to attend a homebirth is unacceptable. Some other form of negligence, for example, failure to diagnose a recognizable high-risk pregnancy, should be necessary for misconduct. Nor is a physician guilty of misconduct in the case of high-risk homebirth when,

<hr/>

[15]*Ibid.*, p. 211. In Jefferson v. Griffin Spalding County Hospital Authority, 247 Ga. 86, 274 S.E.2d 457 (1981), the Georgia Supreme Court upheld a court ordered cesarean delivery, but the delivery was never performed because the condition corrected by itself. This underscores the need for strong proof.

[16]See Edward W. Keyserlingk, "The Unborn Child's Right to Prenatal Care," *Health Law in Canada*, 3, no. 1 (1982), 10–21, and 3, no. 2 (1982), 31–41.

[17]Jane L. Glassco, "Alberta MD's Forbidden to Take Part in Home Births," *The Globe and Mail* (Toronto), May 6, 1981, p. 4.

despite the physician's urgings that the woman go to a hospital, she insists on delivery at home. The choice is between leaving the mother and baby to less adequate care, and perhaps endangering their lives, or attending the birth; it is not acceptable to make the baby pay for its mother's improper conduct. If penalties are to be imposed in such a case, they should be legal ones imposed on the mother, not a danger to the baby's health reinforced by the medical profession.

Case 4.3 Norton Children's Hospitals in Louisville, Kentucky, is the high-risk newborn center for Western Kentucky. In 1978, the obstetrics and gynecology staff agreed that they did not want to serve as the backup hospital for home deliveries. Although no official hospital policy existed, the staff were unanimous; they did not support homebirths, and decided that it was not their role to provide such support. Any physician who wanted to do homebirths should use another hospital for backup. Nonetheless, if someone came to the hospital as a result of complications of a homebirth, the staff would provide treatment.[18]

Here is an informal staff policy discouraging homebirths. But the case is not quite clear, because Norton Children's Hospitals is a high-risk facility to back up other hospitals. Many complications that arise in homebirth do not require a perinatal center; a normal hospital delivery unit will suffice. In this light, Norton Children's ought not be the primary backup hospital for homebirth. Yet, as the only high-risk center for Western Kentucky, it should be willing to handle backup for especially difficult complications for which a regular hospital obstetric unit is inadequate. Unfortunately, the staff had mixed motives: they also wanted to discourage homebirths. The result could simply be worse outcomes for babies.

A closely related question is whether a hospital should refuse privileges to nurse-midwives.[19] The American College of Nurse-Midwives supports practice of nurse-midwives for full delivery in normal pregnancies with physician backup for problems. Sometimes nurse-midwives who want to practice independently and have an arrangement for physician backup are denied hospital privileges. The reasons for such a denial are rather complex, involving such matters as hospital liability and obstetricians' fear of competition. Assuming that the hospital can be protected from liability (for example, by the nurse-midwives paying for extra liability insurance), no sound reason exists to deny hospital privileges to nurse-midwives.

Such a judgment primarily rests on the record of nurse-midwives in providing competent care for normal birth for the last half-century. This extends from the Frontier Nursing Service in the Kentucky hills to practice in birthing centers and hospitals.[20] Nurse-midwives are often preferred by

[18]John Finley, "Delivery Staff Opposes Home-Birth Care," *The Courier-Journal* (Louisville), October 7, 1978, p. A2.

[19]A. Forman and E. Cooper, "Legislation and Nurse-Midwifery Practice in the U.S.A.," *J. Nurse-Midwifery,* 21, no. 2 (1976), 11.

[20]For a good account, see Dorothea Lang, "The American College of Nurse-Midwives (ACNM): What is the Future for Certified Nurse Midwives? In Hospitals? Childbearing Centers? Homebirths?" in *21st Century Obstetrics Now! Vol. 1,* ed. Lee Stewart and David Stewart (Chapel Hill, N.C.: NAPSAC, Inc., 1977), 89–104.

pregnant women; they take more time to explain matters in prenatal visits, provide childbirth preparation classes, and constantly attend the women during labor. They thus establish a better relationship and provide more emotional support and information than do most physicians. Their records for normal deliveries are as good as, or better than, those of the average physician.

In a few states, nurse-midwives are not legally permitted to provide full care for normal pregnancies; and they are not recognized at all in Canada. The long record of adequate care and the obvious satisfaction of many women supports the introduction of policies, regulations, and laws permitting the full practice of nurse-midwifery. Besides, in a country with government health insurance, like Canada, widespread use of nurse-midwives would decrease health care expenditures with no increase in bad outcomes. Physicians could then specialize in the more difficult cases in which their expertise is needed.

One final policy consideration deals with providing facilities for alternative childbirth practices, so that women have the real choice which constitutes a major element in ideal childbirth. Most women might still opt for hospital births, perhaps in hospital birthing centers. In small communities there might be insufficient demand to support such programs. The only way to find out, however, is to adopt policies which at least permit such practices. If the demand does not exist, such practices will not be widely used. If nonstandard hospital childbirth grows, an increase in health risks is unlikely; if risks do increase, the practices can be restricted. At the same time, needless costs for health care might be reduced. Most importantly, the pathological worst-case strategy which now prevails would give way to one that gives women control over the childbirth process that makes it the rewarding experience to which they are ethically entitled.

BIBLIOGRAPHY

HOLMES, HELEN B.; HOSKINS, BETTY B.; and GROSS, MICHAEL, eds. *Birth Control and Controlling Birth: Women-Centered Perspectives*. Clifton, N.J.: The Humana Press, Inc., 1980.

INTERPROFESSIONAL TASK FORCE ON HEALTH CARE OF WOMEN AND CHILDREN *Joint Position Statement on the Development of Family-Centered Maternity/Newborn Care in Hospitals*. Chicago: American College of Obstetricians and Gynecologists, 1978.

KEYSERLINGK, EDWARD W. "The Unborn Child's Right to Prenatal Care," *Health Law in Canada*, 3, 1 (1982), 10–21; and 3, 2 (1982), 31–41.

KITZINGER, SHELIA; and DAVIS, JOHN A., eds. *The Place of Birth*. Oxford: Oxford University Press, 1978.

KLAUS, MARSHALL H.; and KENNELL, JOHN H. *Maternal-Infant Bonding: The Impact of Early Separation or Loss on Family Development*. St. Louis: C. V. Mosby Company, 1976.

ROMALIS, SHELLY, ed. *Childbirth: Alternatives to Medical Control*. Austin: University of Texas Press, 1981.

STEWART, LEE; and STEWART, DAVID, eds. *21st Century Obstetrics Now!* 2 vols. Chapel Hill, N.C.: NAPSAC, Inc., 1977.

CHAPTER 5

Defective Newborns

Despite the availability of genetic screening and high quality childbirth methods, some infants are born with defects. These may be due to genetic conditions, illnesses or drugs taken in pregnancy that have affected the developing fetus, extreme prematurity and low birth weight, or unavoidable damage during delivery. Contemporary neonatal intensive care can save the lives of many such infants who a few decades or even years ago would have had no chance for survival. The great majority of infants treated in neonatal intensive care leave after a few weeks and lead relatively normal lives. Not all are so fortunate. A few have uncorrectable defects or a significant chance of having them, perhaps due to side effects of treatment. Even so, medical treatment can now keep many of these infants alive. Their situations raise some of the most difficult and heart rending issues of human reproduction and bioethics. In this chapter we focus on the difficult and less common cases in which treatment cannot result in a normal healthy child and some significant handicap is inevitable.

Case 5.1 Bernice is delivered at full term weighing 3827 grams (8 lbs. 7 oz.). She has multiple defects, including myelomeningocele (spina bifida) involving a lesion (opening) of the spine of roughly 5 cm. between her shoulder blades; two club feet; and hydrocephalus (a buildup of cerebrospinal fluid in the brain). The thin membrane covering the spinal lesion burst during birth, increasing the chances of infection. Subsequent examination indicates that Bernice has no feeling in her legs. There is also another opening in the spine below the major lesion. The hydrocephalus is not yet severe but it is significant. The lateral ventricles are four to five times normal size, and the upper brain mass is compressed to one-half normal size.

Bernice's prognosis is not good. She will be incontinent, and her legs will be permanently paralyzed. Even with treatment of the hydrocephalus, there is a 70 percent chance that she will have below-average intelligence, and a one-in-three chance that she will be retarded.[1] Aggressive treatment will involve immediate surgery to place a skin graft over the spinal lesion, and in about a week, placement of a shunt to drain fluid from the brain into the abdominal cavity. Further surgery may be required on both feet, the hole at the bottom of the spine, to correct curvature of the spine, and perhaps her bladder and colon. Additional surgery to revise the shunt is also likely. On average, she will require a major operation a year for the first ten to fifteen years of life.

The alternative is to treat only to relieve pain and distress, but not to prolong her life. Infections likely to be lethal will not be treated. The chances are about 50 percent that she will become infected and die within a few months. Most untreated infants like Bernice die within a year, but a few survive longer, sometimes for years. Nontreatment of the hydrocephalus would increase the chances of retardation should she survive, and her head might grow very large.

Bernice's mother, Darlene, is a seventeen-year-old high school dropout. She lives with the father, Charles, a twenty-one-year-old with some college education, but they are not married. Although Charles is employed fulltime, they have little money and no health insurance. At first, both parents hope that some possible treatment will give Bernice a chance for a normal life. When the specialist first informs them that Bernice will be paralyzed and possibly retarded, Darlene becomes upset and has to be given a sedative. Charles does not understand everything the doctor says, but he does say that they do not want Bernice to live paralyzed and retarded. Early the next morning, the doctor visits Darlene and asks whether they want Bernice operated on. The doctor understands her to say they want him to do his best, and schedules surgery, although Darlene thinks she has told him to do what he thinks best. At noon that day Darlene is released from the hospital. She and Charles go to the nursery, and, with tears in their eyes, hold and rock Bernice. They then receive further counseling about Bernice's prospects. The doctor remarks that he personally does not think treatment worthwhile, although he will abide by their wishes. Upon consideration, they decide not to consent to surgery or other life-prolonging treatment. The surgery is cancelled and antibiotics to ward off infection are halted. Charles and Darlene then work out a schedule for going to the hospital each day to feed, diaper, and care for Bernice.

This case raises most of the issues about the care of defective newborns. The basic alternatives in such a case are aggressive treatment to prolong life, involving a long series of operations; or no life-prolonging treatment, only loving care to ward off minor infections and prevent discomfort. Whether one decides on aggressive treatment depends, in the view of many persons, only on the value of life to the infant. Must a decision be based solely on the value of life for the infant, or is it also appropriate to consider the burdens on the parents, siblings, and society? Who should

[1]Leonard Diller, Chester A. Swinyard, and Fred J. Epstein, "Cognitive Function in Children with Spina Bifida," in *Decision Making and the Defective Newborn: Proceedings of a Conference on Spina Bifida and Ethics,* ed. Chester A. Swinyard (Springfield, Ill.: Charles C. Thomas Publisher, 1978), p. 40, Table 3–11.

decide whether or not to give life-prolonging treatment—doctors, parents, courts, or someone else? Should financial considerations be taken into account, either the parents' ability to pay for the treatment or the costs to society if the parents do not or cannot afford to pay?

The Value of Life

Central, but not necessarily conclusive, for any analysis of decisions whether to treat defective newborns is the question of the value of life to the infant. The issue is not the value of the infant's life to others—parents, siblings, or society—but to the infant itself. What conditions make life worth living? Such conditions could range from mere biological life itself, through various capacities of the person, to social factors such as income and living conditions.

Some authors do not ask what makes life worth living, but what makes an infant a person? The general idea is that unless an infant is a person, or at least potentially a person, it has no right to life, and thus nontreatment or perhaps even active killing is permissible. This approach is similar to that used in the abortion controversy about when a fetus has a right to life, although we did not state the issue as "When does a fetus become a person?" Views vary widely as to what factors are relevant to an infant being a person. Some people use relatively stringent requirements so that many infants would not be regarded as persons.[2] Others use much weaker criteria so that only very severely defective infants would not be regarded as persons.[3]

This approach is not acceptable. It radically changes the structure of the question. It becomes, "What kind of being is this?" rather than, "What may or should one ethically do?" Although personhood or moral status may be relevant, it surely does not settle the issue of what one ought to do. We have already seen that a right to life can be ascribed to fetuses at seven months. The personhood approach assumes that having a right to life settles the question of what ought to be done. But the question is whether the right to life should be exercised, whether the life is worth living. To think personhood settles the matter is to confuse the question of what kinds of beings can have a right, with that of whether their lives would have sufficient value to make it worth insisting on that right. It thus implicitly makes the value of life an all-or-nothing matter, and leaves no room for balancing other considerations with it.

The approach used here avoids these problems. We have already asked whether fetuses have moral status. Given that with usual brain functions after seven months they do, their well-being must be considered

[2] Joseph Fletcher, "Indicators of Humanhood: A Tentative Profile of Man," *The Hastings Center Report*, 2, no. 5 (Oct. 1972), 2–4; Joseph Fletcher, "Four Indicators of Humanhood— The Enquiry Matures," *The Hastings Center Report*, 4, no. 6 (Dec. 1974), 4–7.

[3] Eike-Henner W. Kluge, "The Euthanasia of Radically Defective Neonates: Some Statutory Considerations," 6 *Dalhousie L. J.* 229–57 (1980); Paul Ramsey, *Ethics at the Edges of Life* (New Haven and London: Yale University Press, 1978), p. 213; he goes so far as to say anencephalic infants should by definition be said not to have been born alive.

equally with that of adults. However, adults who clearly have moral status (and a right to life) do not always have expectable lives of such value as to make their prolongation advisable. The same conceptual framework applies to infants. One should ask what makes life valuable and whether this infant (or adult) is likely to have a valuable life.

Suggested answers to the question of what makes life valuable resemble those given to the question of when a fetus has moral status. One view is that mere biological life is valuable in itself. Sometimes this view is supported by claims that God has given people life and that it is not appropriately their decision when to end it. But, logically, the claim that God has given life does not entail that it is valuable to the person. One frequently receives gifts for birthdays and other occasions that are not of value to one, except perhaps for the thought that went into them. Moreover, if life were something only God should give or take, it would also be wrong for humans to use medical measures to prolong life. Perhaps God has given life and commands that it be preserved, but then if life is a burden rather than a value to one, one can only conclude that God is malicious.

More seriously, mere biological life is not of value in itself. People in irreversible coma are biologically alive. Whether or not their lives are valuable to others, they surely have no value for themselves. There would be no increase in the value of one's life if two extra years of life in a coma were added at the end. In a coma, one would not experience life at all, and therefore could not experience it as good or bad, as valuable or not.

Views that claim some experiential capacity makes life worth living should also be rejected. Mere experience itself—sentience—does not necessarily have positive value. Life is not necessarily worth living simply because one has sensation, the capacity for interaction with others, or the capacity for thinking. These capacities only indicate that one's life can be of value or disvalue, so that a being with such capacities has moral status; that is, the being's welfare must be considered. For positive value or good, those capacities must be used in ways that bring good experiences—pleasant sensations, loving rather than hateful interactions with others, and pleasant rather than unpleasant or fearful thoughts. This is another reason why the personhood approach is not proper, for it concentrates only on the capacities for experience rather than on the nature of those experiences.

Nevertheless, to the extent one lacks these capacities, one lacks the possibilities for experiences that would make life worth living. If one cannot think, one cannot have the "pleasures" of thinking. If one cannot affectively interact with others, one cannot feel and express love. And if one cannot walk or use one's arms, one cannot have simple pleasures from a walk in the woods or waving to a friend.

The experiences people value in life differ greatly from one individual to another. Some people enjoy eating and others do not. Some people enjoy listening to music, reading, running, and so forth, and others do not. There is no basis for saying that all rational persons would find the same experiences valuable. Which experiences individuals enjoy depends to a large extent on socialization.

The variety of experiences that makes life valuable to people creates little difficulty in deciding whether to prolong the life of adults. Competent adults can decide for themselves whether their expectable life would be valuable to them. Even with previously competent but now incompetent adults, others can reasonably determine from individuals' earlier lives what they found valuable.

With newborn infants, none of this is possible. One must try to decide whether their prospects are such that they will find life valuable. To the extent that they will lack capacities for various types of experiences that many people enjoy, one can conclude that their lives will be less valuable. Even if they have such capacities but will lack social opportunities for the types of experiences many people enjoy, one can reasonably conclude that their lives will be less valuable to them. This last consideration applies to normal as well as abnormal children; we believe that children born to poor, mentally retarded parents are likely to have less valuable lives.

Usually, three factors are used in judging the expectable value of an infant's life to it—mental ability, pain, and physical incapacity. Writers on the subject usually place the greatest emphasis on mental ability. The abilities to think, communicate, and sometimes express love are emphasized. Pain, or the balance of pleasure and pain, receives the second most emphasis. Physical disability is usually treated as of minor concern. In practice, this means that severe retardation is thought to be a strong indication that life would not be of value, whereas paraplegia or even quadriplegia is not usually taken as a strong indication that life would not be valuable.

This ranking and emphasis probably indicates more about the individual and cultural biases of the authors than it does about the value of life. Writers on bioethics are usually intellectuals whose lives revolve around intellectual concerns. Deprive them of this, and their lives might be valueless or miserable. But other people, indeed probably most people, do not live intellectual lives. Physical capacities may be the most important aspect for them. The protagonist in "Whose Life Is It Anyway?" the movie and play about a sculptor who becomes paralyzed below the neck, dramatically illustrates this point. He has above-average intelligence and is not in physical pain, yet he finds the prospect of continued life bad. He can no longer sculpt! He cannot do the things that make life valuable to him. And when it is suggested that he could develop new interests, he rejects the agonizing process involved in destroying his present desires and developing new ones.

In some respects, defective infants may not suffer from mental and physical defects as much as adults who lose capacities, but in other respects they may suffer more. Children who have never been able to walk, for instance, might not develop interests in activities requiring that ability. Children who have been mentally handicapped from birth will not miss the joys of chess, writing, reading Shakespeare, and advanced mathematics. Yet, they might suffer more in other ways. If they are retarded, they might not be able to understand the point of painful treatments, and thus might fear them more. If not retarded, they might be even more acutely aware of physical incapacities and of what they will never be able to do.

All three factors should be taken into account. The relative weights to be assigned to mental and physical activities depend on the cultural environment in which the child would live. The ultimate standard is whether the child will have sufficient capacities and opportunities for fulfilling interests (or desires) and enjoyable experiences to outweigh unfulfilled interests and unpleasant experiences. This standard, unlike the personhood approach, considers opportunities as well as capacities, and emphasizes that these opportunities must offer a balance of good over bad experiences.

These types of considerations can be applied to Bernice. She will be paralyzed from the waist down and cannot have experiences of running, walking, and other such activities. She will have the capacity of sensation, so she can have pleasant and painful experiences. As she will have to undergo many, often painful operations, she will have many unpleasant experiences. The culture of her parents is more physically than intellectually oriented. She will likely have less mental capacity than average and therefore fewer pleasures of thinking, which are apt to loom more important in life for a physically incapacitated person. She might be less able to understand why she is subjected to various painful operations. Given the current provision of social services, she is not likely to have opportunities for many of the enjoyable experiences that she has the capacity to have. Future employment, for example, is doubtful at best. Thus, on the whole, her prospects for a life of value to herself are quite poor, ranging from a minimally valuable life to one that is simply a burden to her. If her lesion had been lower or if she had not had hydrocephalus, her prospects and the likely value of life to her would have been greater.

An objection to this line of argument is that logically one cannot assess the value of lives to others. One cannot have another person's experiences. However, people do in fact make such judgments all the time. Almost anyone of mature years who has lived in society has known some people who lived unhappy, miserable lives, and others who lived relatively happy, enjoyable lives they found worthwhile. These judgments are often confirmed by the individuals themselves. Theoretical accounts of how or why this is may be lacking, but that only shows a defect in theories. People's abilities to judge whether others find their lives valuable vary, but some sensitive people are quite successful at it. Most judgments are of degrees of how good people find their lives, but that does not imply that one cannot also judge when people find their lives, overall, bad.

A second and more common objection is that ethically one should not judge the value of others' lives. To do so is to deny that all lives are equally valuable, to move to a caste, class, or racist system that is antithetical to modern society and values. Often this version of the objection rests on confusing the value of lives to the individuals that live them with their value to others, their social value. To judge by social value would be antithetical to equality and could lead to various injustices, such as saving the life of a miserable banker rather than that of a happy hooker. But the above reasoning was not concerned with social value, only the value to the individuals themselves.

Only four possible approaches to the value of life and treatment decisions exist. (1) The value of life is not considered at all; but this is implausible, for it denies moral consideration and status. (2) More likely, people who claim not to consider the value of life implicitly endorse the second approach: life is assumed to be equally good for all, so all are treated. (3) Life is considered to be equally bad for all infants, so none are treated. No one in fact opts for this possibility. (4) The last approach is to make selective decisions to treat on the basis of the likelihood that the infants will live lives they find valuable.

The second approach treats all infants equally. However, it may be wrong to do so, for not all lives may be worth living. There is almost certainly a built-in set of incorrect outcomes or errors, namely, all those cases that are treated in which the lives subsequently are not found valuable. Moreover, the notion of equality involved is that everyone gets the same thing; equality consists of giving life-prolonging treatment to everyone.

The last approach also runs the risks of incorrect outcomes of errors, both of not treating some cases that should be treated and of treating others that ought not, as judged by the value of the lives that would have been or are lived by the individuals. There is no reason to believe that more errors will result with this approach than with the second. One could only reach that conclusion if one believed that life is valuable no matter what the experiences involved. Of course, some errors can be worse than others. Many people believe that an error that ends a life found to be of value is worse than an error that prolongs a life found to be of disvalue. But there is no logical basis for the belief. Depriving someone of a good is certainly not worse than imposing an equal harm.

One can consider the probability of errors in either direction and the amount of harm likely from each. One can then make one's treatment decisions so as to minimize the overall harm from errors. In doing so, for spina bifida cases, one must consider that some untreated infants will survive and will probably have greater handicaps than they would have were they treated. Such a consideration suggests that a selective treatment policy should be conservative with respect to nontreatment.

Such a selective nontreatment policy is acceptable. The concept of equality underlying it is equality of consideration. People do not automatically receive the same thing—life-prolonging treatment—but they do receive equal consideration as to whether their lives are likely to be valuable to them. Nonselective treatment ignores the likely value of life to individuals. It fails to consider the differences among persons. At its core, it lacks the humanity that considers differences between individuals and the differences in the likely value of their lives to them. It treats persons like interchangeable parts in a machine.

Decisions Not to Treat

Regardless of their views about the value of life, in two types of cases almost everyone agrees that nontreatment is appropriate. In these types of cases, treatment is futile or pointless. The first type involves an infant who has an overwhelming defect or defects. The most commonly cited example is an infant who is anencephalic, that is, born with no upper brain. Such an infant can never have significant awareness; it even lacks the capacities for moral status. Even the strongest advocates of aggressive treatment do not treat such infants.

The second category of infants is those who are dying and can only have the process prolonged. Disagreement can arise about the borders of this category. Still, some infants are undergoing an irreversible degenerative process which treatment can only retard or arrest for a brief period of time.

Since death will come in a relatively short time whether or not they are treated, no one seriously advocates prolonging the dying process by a few hours or days. Disagreement arises when it is a question of adding weeks or perhaps months of life.

Bernice in Case 5.1 does not fall into either of these categories. She is not dying. Given treatment, there is a good chance that she will live for years. Without treatment, her chances of living even one year are very poor. A decision not to treat in cases like Bernice's rests significantly on judgments about the value of her expectable life, because unlike the previous types of cases, treatment can significantly extend conscious life.

In cases of this sort, perhaps the most central issue is whether any considerations other than the expectable value of life to the infant can ethically be taken into account. In particular, can the effects her continued living will have on her parents and society be considered, or must an ethical decision depend solely on the value of life to her? If effects on others can be considered, then sometimes different decisions will result. First, an infant might have expectable life of minimum value to it, but the burdens on others might be such as to tip the scales toward nontreatment. Second, an infant might have an expectable quality of life that would not be of value to it, but benefits to others might be sufficient to tip the scales in favor of treatment. Although this sort of situation is not one that many people worry about, it can arise when physicians treat in order to learn more about the various possible forms of treatment. An infant might be kept alive for the benefit of experimentation rather than the value of life to it.[4]

One approach is to bring these other factors into account, but only insofar as they affect the value of an infant's life to it. For example, it has been suggested that the quality (or value) of an infant's life depends on the infant's natural endowment or capacities as affected by the expectable contributions from home and society.[5] This type of analysis for determining an infant's value of life is appropriate. As noted, it is not merely having capacities that counts, but the experiences that result from their use. The character of such experiences undoubtedly depends to a large extent on contributions from family and society. Nonetheless, this approach does not really consider the possible benefits and burdens to others of the infant's continued life. Even though contributions from a poor family might be low, and the burden on the family great, this approach does not examine the burden as such.

The primary concern in the literature has not been that the infants' lives would lack value because others could or would not assist them, but that infants with prospects for lives valuable to them might not be treated because of their burden on others. In effect, the social value of infants would be taken into account. Were the value negative (a burden), they would not be treated. Many people believe that the well-being of the infants should be the sole consideration. Otherwise, they claim, infants would be denied an equal claim to a valuable life and be used as mere means to others' ends.

---

[4]For an account of a case that appears to partly involve this, see Robert Stinson and Peggy Stinson, "On the Death of a Baby," *Atlantic Monthly* (July 1979), 64–72.

[5]Anthony Shaw, "Who Should Die and Who Should Decide," in *Infanticide and the Value of Life,* ed. Marvin Kohl (Buffalo, N.Y.: Prometheus Books, 1978), p. 105.

They reject any moral principle that sacrifices the lives of some because they are a burden to others.

Considering the effects on others of the continued life of infants does not deny them an equal claim to a valuable life. The infants' claim to life can be considered; taking account of the burdens of others is giving equal consideration to the claims of others to a valuable life. To ignore such effects amounts to denying consideration of the value of their lives to them. Granted, the lives of others are not at stake, but their value is. Moreover, one cannot claim that life itself for one person always outweighs considerations of its value to others, without returning to the unacceptable claim that life itself, regardless of the kinds of experiences involved, is ultimately of value. The value of the continued existence of a person is the value of that life to the person, except for the social value, which is in dispute. The choice is simply between value in the life of one person and value in the lives of others.

Nor is it clear that infants would be used as means for the ends of others. The classic formulation of the ethical principle about treating people as means states that persons must not be treated as *mere* means, that is, for ends they cannot also share.[6] If an infant were capable of and voluntarily chose nontreatment to spare others, the infant would not be used as a mere means. The difficulty is that an infant is incapable of making such a judgment or choice. Either the whole concept of treating as a mere means vanishes because there is no way to make sense of an infant sharing an end, or else one must attribute some reasonable ends to the infant. Only treating infants in ways incompatible with reasonably attributed ends then constitutes treating them as a mere means. To claim that depriving an infant of any life of minimally positive value always treats the infant as a mere means amounts to attributing pure self-interestedness to the infant. One presupposes that the infant could never reasonably have the well-being of others as an end. One could equally reasonably assume that an infant would have a concern for others, especially its parents, and could share in the end of losing a life of minimal value to avoid suffering and burdens of its parents. No persuasive reason presents itself for making one assumption rather than the other. Consequently, this argument is inconclusive.

Finally, the claim that considering effects on others means sacrificing the lives of some because they are a burden on others primarily restates the previous arguments. It assumes that life itself takes precedence over other considerations, or that nontreatment is using infants as mere means for others. Perhaps the use of the word 'sacrifice' makes this claim seem compelling. One often thinks of sacrifice as actively killing. A principle that it is permissible to sacrifice (kill) another person (a boss or in-law) because he or she is a burden is unacceptable. But in the sort of cases under consideration one is really faced with some sacrifice, however one decides. Either an infant sacrifices a life of minimal value to it, or parents or others sacrifice some experiences that would make their lives valuable. Someone loses for the sake of another; the questions are who loses, what, and how much.

The positive argument for considering burdens on others is quite

---

[6]Immanuel Kant, *The Moral Law: Kant's Groundwork of the Metaphysics of Morals,* tr. H. J. Paton (New York: Barnes & Noble, Inc., 1963), p. 96; Akademie, page 429.

simple. In almost all areas of life, the effects of conduct on everyone are relevant to whether the conduct is right or wrong. In short, a basic ethical consideration in evaluating conduct is its effect on everyone affected. Few ethical theories have ever denied this relevance. Only in particular contexts where competing considerations have already been weighed and taken into account in formulating moral principles are effects on others ignored. For example, a lawyer assigned by a court to defend a person accused of an especially heinous crime ought not consider the effects of doing so on himself or herself. But this point results from a previous weighing of the effects on everyone of having a rule entitling all criminal defendants to legal counsel, the lawyer's voluntary decision to enter the field, and the likely effects on the lawyer. Were doing so likely to destroy the lawyer's practice or life, a judge would and should allow the lawyer to withdraw from the case.

Consequently, the burden to others of prolonging the life of a seriously defective infant is a relevant consideration. We saw in Chapter 2 that the burden on others is a relevant reason for not bringing an unborn child into existence. This principle can now be reformulated as follows: The burden to others is a reason not to bring a child into existence or to prolong a child's existence. This must be weighed against other reasons, in particular the value of life of an existing child. Consequently, this principle must be used carefully in decisions not to treat. It should be used only when the value of life to the child is questionable, because the burdens on others are likely to concern matters of lesser importance for a valuable life. Should the burdens on parents be too great, but the child's life reasonably be one of value, the parents can relinquish their rights to the child. While this might be a significant blow to the parents, the harm to them would be less than the loss of a reasonably valuable life to the infant. But because relinquishing custody of a child is usually a burden to parents, one cannot ethically require them to relinquish the child whenever its life might be of minimal value to it. One would then be causing the parents a greater burden than the benefit being gained.

Thus the value of an infant's life to it is the first and primary consideration in deciding not to treat, but at least in close cases the burdens on the parents and others may be sufficient to weigh the decision in favor of nontreatment. In Bernice's case, her life would probably not have value for her, but this would partly depend on whether she was mentally handicapped, and on the degree of the handicap. Considering the low income and youth of Charles and Darlene, they will not be capable of making large contributions to Bernice's life. So the chances that Bernice's life will be of significant value to her are minimal. People who have survived with such defects generally agree that one should not treat an infant severely affected with myelomeningocele.[7] Thus, it would not be necessary to consider the burdens on the parents, Charles and Darlene, in order to reach a decision not to treat. If such considerations were necessary, the burdens of lifelong care on a couple with such limited resources would be devastating, and tip the decision to nontreatment.

---

[7]John Lorber, "Discussion," in *Decision Making and the Defective Newborn: Proceedings of a Conference on Spina Bifida and Ethics,* ed. Chester A. Swinyard (Springfield, Ill.: Charles C. Thomas Publisher, 1978), p. 248.

Finally, the principle of burdens to others does not support experimental treatment of infants with miserable lives. The principle only states that burdens, not benefits, to others are to be considered. Rational persons might accept a principle permitting the infliction of torture or a miserable existence on one person for the benefit of others in extremely rare and exceptional circumstances, but they would not accept this for very common circumstances, as in neonatal care. Such treatment violates the fundamental right not to be caused unnecessary suffering, a right that fetuses acquire at about five months gestation. Such experimental treatment is not necessary. Many infants born with defects should be treated without consideration of benefits to others from experimentation. In their cases, the research might be beneficial to them. In this regard, it should be noted that most treatment of seriously defective or ill newborns is almost by definition experimental care.[8] In the case of infants better not treated because their lives would be bad, treatment, even if "successful," would be not a benefit but a harm. It would prolong a miserable existence. Treatment techniques can be improved by experimentation on infants who would benefit. In the future these techniques can be used on infants who previously would not have been treated, but they may then be used because, with treatment, they now have a reasonable chance for a valuable life. That is, successful experimentation on spina bifida infants who are not as damaged as Bernice may improve techniques so that in the future, infants with her condition would, with treatment, have a chance of a valuable life.

Who Decides?

Even if it is acceptable to treat defective newborns selectively and to take into account the burdens of their survival on others, one must still determine who should make treatment decisions. A variety of people have been suggested—physicians, parents, ethics committees, and courts. In current practice, the choice basically boils down to either physicians or parents, because most hospitals do not even have ethics committees and the court system is unprepared to provide decisions for all such cases. Nevertheless, not all decisions need to be made by the same people, so limited roles for committees and courts are possible. Determining their role is primarily a policy matter.

Ethical Analysis

The decision-maker principles developed in the previous chapter are relevant here. Those principles indicate that decisions should be made by persons who have special expertise or who will bear most of the consequences. The choice between physicians and parents rests on these factors.

The reasons for physicians making the decisions are primarily these: They have expertise concerning likely outcomes; parents are not capable of

[8]Albert R. Jonsen and George Lister, "Newborn Intensive Care: The Ethical Problems," *The Hastings Center Report*, 8, no. 1 (Feb. 1978), 16–17.

Defective Newborns **99**

making reasonable decisions; and should the decision be against treatment, parents would be relieved of any guilt for the death of an infant. The claim of expertise is countered by the argument that decisions not to treat are essentially based on values and ethics; about these, physicians can claim no special expertise. Their information about outcomes could be given to others. Parents' ability to make reasonable decisions is considered below. Whether physicians should relieve parents of possible guilt depends on whether parents are capable of handling such feelings. Of course, if parents make a proper decision, they have no rational grounds for guilt, but inappropriate guilt can be as psychologically burdensome as appropriate guilt. Against physicians' making the decisions is the claim that they do not have to bear the major consequences.

The major argument in favor of parents making the decision is that they will bear the consequences. They must bear lifelong care of a handicapped child, the death of their child, or the pangs of relinquishing it to another. However, a number of objections are made against decisions made by parents. These objections either do not arise for parental childbirth decisions or are more serious for nontreatment decisions. The first objection is that parents will be biased against treatment. In childbirth, their primary motivations are psychologically rewarding experiences that closely involve the infant, as in bonding, and so are beneficial for the infant as well as the parents. In decisions about treatment of defective newborns, the interests of parents and infants are not so parallel. Treatment of infants, even if it provides a valuable life, will impose a tremendous burden on the parents, psychologically, socially, and financially. Given this fundamental conflict of interest, the objectors conclude, parents are not the appropriate decision makers.

Parents do have many interests contrary to those of a defective infant. But how likely are these interests to influence parental decisions improperly? If it was a planned pregnancy, parents have begun to develop a love for the child. Maternal-infant attachment usually begins in the later stages of pregnancy. If in the first day after birth they are permitted to hold or at least touch the infant, bonding is apt to develop rather strongly. Before they made the decision not to treat, both Charles and Darlene held Bernice in their arms. It was a moment of love, not self-interested concern. Moreover, the love of parents grows when they continue to care for children after a decision not to treat. The first concern expressed by most parents is for their child.

Other people might also be biased. Physicians might worry about whether they will be paid, about spending hours in treating near-hopeless cases, and about the general burden on society. Judges and members of committees might also have other concerns, such as their reputations. Treatment of any severely damaged newborn is likely to involve a social cost that will fall on all taxpayers. Although this cost to any one individual will be small and thus perhaps not likely to affect a decision, so might also be the person's love or concern for the infant.

A second reason against parents making treatment decisions is that they may not understand the options. Treatment decisions for defective newborn infants involve matters more complex than most decisions about childbirth. For example, in cases like Bernice's, parents may not understand that surgery will not correct the paralysis; the nature of the spinal lesion which makes correction impossible; and the implications of a shunt for hydrocephalus.

Nonetheless, parents can come to grasp the fundamentals of the options, but this will require more than two half-hour discussions with a physician. The first conversation hits parents such a blow—being told that their baby will be paralyzed and possibly retarded—that little else can be absorbed. They are not ready, by a second conversation the next morning, to make a decision. Instead, many hours of counseling spaced out over several days are needed. With such counseling and an explanation in terms that a layperson can understand, most parents can grasp the fundamental choice before them. After all, to make a decision in spina bifida cases, they do not need to know precisely which vertebrae and nerves are involved, or how cerebrospinal fluid is produced.

A third reason against parents making these decisions is that they are too emotionally distraught to think clearly. Of course, they are emotionally distraught. They have lost the normal baby they wanted and expected. But, a good deal of the emotional stress is due to their love of the infant. If they did not care for the infant, they would be less upset. It is not obvious that persons under appropriate emotional stress (that based upon reality rather than neurotic or psychotic reactions) cannot make the reasonable decisions. In other aspects of life—divorce, business, combat—people sometimes make reasonable decisions when emotionally distraught. Thus, we can conclude that with appropriate counseling, many parents are capable of making reasonable decisions about treatment.[9]

Case 5.2 Earl is born with Down syndrome and duodenal atresia (a blockage preventing food passing from the stomach into the intestine). Surgery for duodenal atresia is a fairly routine operation for infants. With surgery, Earl can be expected to live a reasonably long life, but due to Down syndrome, he will be retarded. The degree of retardation is unpredictable, varying from profound in a few such infants to moderate or mild in others. Most people with Down syndrome are loveable, pleasant, and trainable. If the surgery is not performed, then Earl will die unless fed intravenously, because he is unable to take food by mouth.

In such cases, parents are almost evenly divided about whether to treat, about half opting for treatment and half not.[10] Thus, some people object to parents making decisions because infants with essentially similar conditions may or may not be treated, may live or die, depending on parental choices.[11] Indeed, it appears to depend simply on whether the parents want the child. This, it is objected, is unjust; medically similar cases are not treated the same.

[9]See Raymond S. Duff, "Counseling Families and Deciding Care of Severely Defective Children: A Way of Coping with 'Medical Vietnam'," *Pediatrics*, 67, no. 3 (1981), 316.

[10]D. P. Girvan and C. A. Stephens, "Congenital Intrinsic Duodenal Obstruction," *J. Ped. Surg.*, 9 (1974), 833–39; cited in Anthony Shaw, "Who Should Die and Who Should Decide," p. 104.

[11]See Richard Sherlock, "Selective Non-Treatment of Newborns," *Journal of Medical Ethics*, 5, no. 3 (1979), 139.

This objection involves two separate claims—that it is wrong for infants with similar medical conditions to be treated differently, and that allowing parents to make decisions results in such differential treatment. The differential treatment of infants with similar medical conditions results partly from the importance of possible social and parental contributions for the likely value of life to infants. If possible social and parental support varies, so will the likely value of life for medically similar cases. In the more difficult cases with which we are primarily concerned, differences will also result from varying evaluations of possible outcomes. This latter feature is also an acceptable basis for variable treatment in borderline cases. Consequently, different treatment in medically similar cases is not necessarily unjust or unethical. Indeed, when the value of life will differ significantly (from good to bad), similar treatment would be unjust. Perhaps different treatment seems wrong because we say an infant was not treated because its parents did not want it. Yet, often this means that the parents did not want the infant to suffer what they think would have been a bad life or a life of no value for the infant.

Consequently, it is not necessarily allowing parents to make such decisions that produces the different treatment decisions for similar medical conditions. If physicians or anyone else were to make the decisions and consider social factors affecting the value of an infant's life, they also would arrive at different decisions for infants with similar medical conditions. Even if social factors are not taken into account, different decisions are made by different physicians. They disagree to some extent in their medical prognoses and evaluations of what type of life is valuable. Thus, if physicians make decisions, although the patients of each physician are treated more or less the same, differences exist among physicians. If parents make the decisions, decisions vary among the patients of each physician. About the same number of cases are likely to be treated or not whether physicians or patients make decisions. If different physicians made decisions in cases like that of Earl (Case 5.2), perhaps about half of them would treat and half would not.[12] Variability of treatment is acceptable only because differences in social or parental support significantly affect the value of life, or because the case is a borderline one where burdens to others make a difference. These features can change over time so that cases that were previously borderline no longer are. Children like Earl provide an example of this. Until the 1970s, social provisions and care for people with Down syndrome were not very good. Governmental services were often poor and children were often "warehoused" in large, underfunded, state institutions. During the last decade or so these conditions have changed significantly. Medical developments, such as early stimulation programs, also improve outcomes. Consequently, the prospects of a valuable life for children with Down syndrome have increased significantly. What once were borderline or close cases no longer are.

Thus, when the likely value of life to infants is questionable, parents should make decisions for or against life-prolonging treatment of their chil-

---

[12]See David Todres, "Discussion," in *Decision Making and the Defective Newborn: Proceedings of a Conference on Spina Bifida and Ethics,* ed. Chester H. Swinyard (Springfield, Ill.; Charles C. Thomas Publisher, 1978), p. 232. Approximately one-third would treat and two-thirds would not for cases like Bernice's in 5.1; *ibid.,* p. 231.

dren. Many are capable, with adequate counseling, of doing so. They bear more of the consequences than other possible decision makers. Decisions will vary in medically similar cases, but that can ethically result from different social and parental contributions to the expectable value of life to the infant, differences in burdens to others, and differences in evaluations of the value of life.

Policy Analysis

The objections to decisions made by parents because they are biased, emotionally distraught, and lack understanding do require some policy considerations to limit parental decision making. In practice, physicians control parental decision making in the sense of keeping it within limits. Some keep it within what they think is an acceptable range, and some subtly or unsubtly control the parents so that the decision is that which the doctors think best. There are good policy reasons for such control, even if some physicians use it to give only the appearance of parental decision making.

In a few cases, parents will be incapable of making reasonable decisions. If parents are deciding without any significant consideration for the infant, or lack understanding of the essential elements of the choice, or are too distraught to think clearly, they should not be making the decision. By talking to parents, physicians and counselors should be able to determine whether any of these conditions obtains. For example, if parents were to talk only about how they will ever manage or how caring for the infant will disrupt their lives, then their bias is dominating the decision making and they should not be deciding. The objection is not that they will make the wrong decision, but that they are not capable of making a rational decision.

Although parents should not be making decisions if any of these three conditions pertains, in practice nothing needs to be done unless they are making an obviously wrong decision. Suppose parents decide not to treat, primarily from considerations of themselves, but in fact such a decision is appropriate even when the value of life for the infant is given primary importance. Then physicians or others need not intervene. If parents are simply too distraught to make any decision, a physician can usually make the decision; such parents usually go along with what the physician recommends.

Occasionally, a parental decision will be clearly wrong and the parents will insist on their course of action. If parents refuse to permit treatment in cases that clearly should be treated, for example, do not want to feed an infant with Down syndrome but no other anomaly, physicians can go to court and have the child removed from the parents' custody. Thus, courts do have a function of controlling decisions when they are clearly wrong. Courts make these decisions on the basis of the infant's best interests. And as argued above, the expectable value of life to the infant is the primary consideration, but not the only one. Consequently, the courts should intervene only when the value of life to the infant clearly outweighs possible burdens to others. Otherwise, they should leave the decision to parents. In general, courts are likely to make decisions primarily on the basis of medical criteria. Thus, the trend of decisions has been to order treatment for cases like that of Earl.[13] This trend has not yet been unanimous, but the general improvement of prospects for such children noted above does make it appropriate. However, one must not go from these situations to supporting treatment for all Down syndrome infants, no matter what other conditions they suffer.

This latter possibility has been raised by regulations of the U.S. Department of Health and Human Services. A 1982 case like that of Earl in which parents elected nontreatment and courts upheld their decision prompted the Department to respond. It sent a letter to all hospitals indicating that federal funds could be withheld should hospitals fail to treat if "(1) the withholding is based on the fact that the infant is handicapped; and (2) the handicap does not render the treatment or nutritional sustenance medically contraindicated."[14]

There are a number of problems with this regulation. First, the substantive principle is either trivial or unacceptable.[15] It is trivial if one emphasizes withholding due to handicap, because the reason for withholding treatments concerns the value of expectable life, not the handicap itself. It is unacceptable if "medically contraindicated" is taken literally, for there are no medical reasons which make surgery in cases of Down syndrome, spina bifida, or most other defects medically inappropriate. The expectable value of life should ethically be considered in such decisions and sometimes make treatment inappropriate. This regulation seems to ignore that.

Second, and more to the point of our present concern with who decides, federal regulation by withholding funds can cause confusion and place hospitals and physicians in a "no-win" position. The problem is that a conflict can arise between state law and federal regulations, with physicians and hospitals caught in between. In the case that prompted the letter, state courts upheld the parental decision. Physicians cannot legally operate without parental or court permission. Yet, the federal government could disagree and cut off funds to the hospital for not operating. Such a situation is unacceptable. Consequently, the federal government should cut off funds only in cases in which physicians do not appeal to a court for a permission to operate which they clearly would have received.

Courts should be able both to order treatment when parents do not want it, and to stop it when parents do want it but it is causing an infant pointless suffering. No direct case of the latter sort seems to have occurred.[16] Physicians can more easily restrain parents from treatment and are more willing to go along with requests for treatment even though they personally disagree. Physicians can prevent parents opting for treatment when it is not appropriate, such as anencephalic infants, by simply not presenting it as an option.

[13]See *In re* B, (1981) 1 W.L.R. 1421.

[14]Rehabilitation Act of 1973, 29 U.S.C. 794, section 504. See "Notice to Health Care Providers," *The Hastings Center Report,* 12, no. 4 (August 1982), 6.

[15]See Norman Fost, "Putting Hospitals on Notice," *The Hastings Center Report,* 12, no. 4 (August 1982), 5–8; Robert M. Veatch, "Severe Handicaps Raise Major Issues of Medical Ethics," *The Seattle Times,* August 22, 1982, p. A19.

[16]The courts did refuse permission for physicians to treat a sixty-seven year old, profoundly retarded man for leukemia; Superintendent of Belchertown State School v. Saikewicz, 373 Mass. 728, 370 N.E.2d 417 (1977).

They can merely say, "There is nothing that can be done." Too often this is done when plausible treatment is available at regional centers, and the result is children who survive with greater handicaps than they would otherwise have had. Again, this method should only be used when, on the basis of the best available medical information, treatment would clearly be inappropriate. Because physicians have been trained to preserve life, often they are willing to try treatment even though it appears pointless, and so they do not restrain parents. Sometimes such treatment is provided for a day or two while the parents come to realize that treatment is inappropriate. This approach applies to infants who are dying. It does not work well with infants who are not dying, like Bernice in Case 5.1; once her back has been closed and a shunt installed, her life has probably been ensured for a while—until infection or shunt blockage.

Thus, as a matter of actual practice, parents are allowed to make decisions whether to treat. If physicians strongly disagree with parental decisions not to treat, then courts can and do make decisions, primarily based on the expectable value of life to the infant. Hospitals or physicians exercise control over those cases that clearly should not be treated by not offering treatment as a choice. One should not ignore this point. In effect, parents have discretion only within limits. Some cases, according to the best information, clearly should not be treated, and in those cases parents are not and should not be given an option to treat. Other cases clearly should be treated, and if parents do not want treatment, courts should order it in the best interests of the infant. This is an acceptable allocation of decision making. No one is given complete control over the life and death of another to be exercised without any protections against arbitrary and improper decisions.

Better to Kill?

If a decision is made not to treat an infant, then would it not be better simply to kill the infant? In a famous case similar to Earl's (5.2) at Johns Hopkins Hospital, after a decision was made not to treat the intestinal blockage, the infant was left to die unfed and minimally attended. It took fifteen days before he died of dehydration and starvation. In such cases, since the decision has been made that the infant should not live, would it not be more humane to end the life easily and quickly by administering a lethal injection? The infant as well as the nursing staff and parents would be spared suffering. And in cases like that of Bernice in 5.1, the process may be much more drawn-out. One is in effect waiting for a lethal infection or some other lethal condition to develop. Some such infants live many months.

Ethical Analysis

This issue is usually stated as a choice between active and passive euthanasia. Active euthanasia is the deliberate killing of a person for that person's benefit, while passive euthanasia is allowing a person to die by not providing life-prolonging treatment. Most of the discussion in the literature has focused on how active and passive euthanasia can or should be distinguished conceptually and whether there is an intrinsic moral difference between the two.

It is quite difficult to state an acceptable theoretical distinction between active and passive euthanasia. One difficulty is that it is not simply a difference between doing and not doing something. Turning off a respirator is doing something, but it is classified as passive euthanasia. Perhaps the underlying conceptual difference is that in passive euthanasia the person dies from a disease or defect which is allowed to cause death, whereas in active euthanasia it is not the disease or defect that causes death but a chain of events initiated by the person performing it, as by a lethal injection. A further conceptual difficulty is that one cannot easily distinguish these causes. If causes are necessary conditions without which something would not have occurred, then failing to provide treatment is such a necessary condition and a cause of death. (Failure to provide treatment is a legal cause only if there is a duty to provide the treatment.)

Whatever the difficulties in conceptually distinguishing active and passive euthanasia, operationally the differences are clear. Not providing treatment, such as the operations in Cases 5.1 and 5.2, or withdrawing treatments already started, such as antibiotics or life support systems, constitutes passive euthanasia. Giving overdoses of morphine or injections of potassium chloride are active euthanasia. For almost any proposed action with respect to a defective infant, few people would have any difficulty classifying it as passive or active euthanasia.

Some people believe that active euthanasia is never morally justifiable but passive euthanasia may be, while others believe that both may be justifiable in some situations but that it is more difficult to justify active than passive euthanasia, that is, that it takes stronger reasons to justify it. If there is such a difference in all cases, it must be due to some morally important feature that differs between killing and allowing to die.

Many philosophers deny that there is any intrinsic moral difference between killing (active euthanasia) and allowing to die (passive euthanasia). Such a claim must be carefully understood. It applies only to cases in which the motive, intention, and consequences are the same. If two people act from the same motive (such as to spare an infant suffering a miserable life), intend death, and the consequences are the same (for example, a quick death), it is ethically irrelevant whether their conduct constitutes active or passive euthanasia. Even if this claim is correct, it is rarely directly relevant to clinical situations because the consequences of active and passive euthanasia are almost always different. This does not, however, constitute an argument for the preferability of passive over active euthanasia. The consequences of passive euthanasia might be worse than those of active euthanasia. Indeed, that is the pull of the Johns Hopkins case where, once a decision not to treat was made, active euthanasia of the infant seemed preferable for all concerned, except perhaps a person who had to carry it out.

The primary difference between active and passive euthanasia in most practical situations is that with passive euthanasia it will be longer before the infant dies, if it does. In a case like Bernice's, death is unlikely to result for days, months, perhaps years following a decision not to treat. Had active euthanasia been used, death would have resulted very quickly. Consequently, in evaluating active and passive euthanasia, one should focus on the extra time before death in passive euthanasia, because that will be important whatever the intrinsic similarity or difference between active and passive euthanasia.

Much depends on what happens during this time. Here it is useful to contrast a case like Bernice's with that of the infant with Down syndrome and intestinal blockage at Johns Hopkins. In cases like Bernice's, the infant is given loving care by the parents, who hold, feed, cuddle, diaper, and spend much time with their baby. It is likely that infants are comforted by such care. They will not feel much pain, for pain medication will be provided. When they die, their parents can grieve for them and feel that they have given them loving care. In the Johns Hopkins case, the parents never came to see their baby after making the decision not to treat. Nor did the nursing staff give much loving care; the infant was not to be fed, so it received only routine diapering and other services.

The time parents spend with their infant is emotionally important to the parents and probably to the child. It enables parents to come to accept the death, even though they develop stronger ties with the infant than they would otherwise. What was so grossly wrong in the Johns Hopkins case was not that the infant was allowed to die rather than be killed, but rather how the infant was allowed to die. Its rejection by parents and nursing and medical staff gave evidence of, and helped to develop, disrespect for infants. This attitude, as expressed in the conduct of the case, undoubtedly caused extra suffering for the nursing staff who were trained and disposed to provide loving care for severely damaged newborn infants. It was contrary to the emotional tenor of a neonatal intensive care unit. Consequently, if the time an infant lives while being allowed to die is well spent in loving care by parents and staff, this period is beneficial for all concerned. Passive euthanasia in such circumstances is thus preferable to active euthanasia.

This does not mean that active euthanasia would always be unacceptable. For example, if an infant is in uncontrollable pain, or so drugged to prevent pain that no interaction between infant and parents is possible, or has so little time left that loving care is hardly possible, then active euthanasia might have the same consequences. However, in those cases, death is likely to ensue in a brief period of time, and the choice between active and passive euthanasia is practically insignificant as to consequences. Moreover, if such a situation were to develop after a period of loving care, active euthanasia might cause psychological difficulties for the parents, even if there is no ethical basis for guilt or refusal to acquiesce in active euthanasia.

This leaves one type of situation in which active euthanasia might be more humane; but even there, active euthanasia faces significant objections which limit it. Suppose, as occasionally happens, an infant like Bernice lives for six months or a year and is severely retarded. There is still no prospect of alleviating the underlying conditions of paralysis and retardation. Perhaps at some point the emotional drain on parents and staff would be so great that active euthanasia might be appropriate. Even then, that might be the wrong course. If such an infant survives six months and its health is good enough that it is likely to survive for some time, perhaps treatment should be started.[17] Indeed, after a few weeks in which bonding has occurred, many parents request aggressive treatment. Such an option would never arise if active euthanasia had been practiced. A passive approach allows for mistaken diagnoses or prognoses to be realized and changes of mind to occur. A similar approach can be used for highly premature infants, but for them one waits only a couple of days to determine how the infants are likely to do.

Policy Analysis

At present, active euthanasia is illegal in the United States, Canada, and most of the world. One must take this factor into account. Physicians or parents who practiced active euthanasia would be liable to criminal sanctions, although very few such cases have been prosecuted, even fewer have resulted in convictions, and heavy sentences are rarely, if ever, given. Thus, active euthanasia is almost certainly unethical as long as these laws remain. The policy question is whether active euthanasia should be legalized for specific situations. In particular, the concern here is whether it should be legalized for defective children, whatever might be the case for adults.

Perhaps the best proposal for legalization of active euthanasia of such infants is that drafted by Arval A. Morris. His proposal would legalize active euthanasia for children under eighteen years of age who have an irremediable condition that renders the child "incapable of the rational or functional existence needed to enjoy the most minimal amount of human goods necessary to constitute ordinary human life in its most minimal sense" or "of leading a rational existence."[18] Before euthanasia may be administered, there must be written consent from the parents and approval by an ethics committee of seven persons from diverse backgrounds. The committee must have determined upon full evidence (including diagnoses of two physicians) that active euthanasia would be in the best interests of the child. Medical personnel, who act in good faith reliance on written consent of the parents and approval of the committee, are protected from liability.

A number of objections can be made to such a proposal. First, despite the careful protections involved in it, the procedure might be inappropriately used. Mistakes can be made. The proposal seems to recognize this by containing a clause protecting medical personnel from liability when acting on a good faith belief that they have appropriate authorization. A good faith belief is not the same as actually having the authority. Also, an unscrupulous physician might not provide completely accurate information to the committee. Second, mistaken diagnoses are possible. With newborn infants it is usually quite difficult to determine the degree of mental retardation, and that is central to whether or not infants will have a rational existence. Third, the proposal assumes that medical personnel will administer lethal injections. It might be very difficult to get physicians or nursing staff to do

[17]John Lorber, "Ethical Problems in the Management of Myelomeningocele and Hydrocephalus—2," *Nursing Times*, March 25, 1976, p. 9.

[18]Arval A. Morris, "Proposed Legislation," in *Infanticide and the Value of Life,* ed. Marvin Kohl (Buffalo, N.Y.: Prometheus Books, 1978), p. 222.

so. Moreover it might be very bad for health care personnel to take life.[19] All their training is directed toward preserving life, and such a change might weaken their general dedication to preserving life. It could cause psychological and emotional difficulties for individuals practicing active euthanasia.

As we saw, passive euthanasia is usually better for the parents and infants because of the time it allows for loving care. Nevertheless, some infants do survive, often for years, without any rational capabilities and with severe physical handicaps. A tiny majority have severely crippling and painful conditions and are so retarded they cannot speak. In these exceedingly rare cases, active euthanasia might be acceptable. To prolong their existence is to prolong pointless suffering, and is contrary to their interests.

A modified version of Morris's proposal might be acceptable for these rare cases. First, experience with committees that authorize sterilization of retarded persons has shown that often they provide little protection and scrutiny. As the number of such cases should be quite small, it would be better to have a judicial determination in each case. This would not constitute a burden on the courts and would provide extra protection. It would prevent very rapid decisions, but active euthanasia is best reserved for cases in which the child is likely to live and suffer for a long time. Second, such a measure should be restricted to infants over a year old. That time is needed to ensure diagnosis of eventual deficits, especially mental deficit. Third, specific individuals might be designated to carry out active euthanasia. This would relieve physicians and other health care personnel of the burden of conflicting sentiments and psychological problems.

Finally, although burden to others is ethically relevant in decisions whether to treat, Morris is correct not to allow such considerations in decisions about active euthanasia. To do so would open the door to placing too much emphasis on social value. Candidates would probably be in institutions, so the parental burden of their continued existence should not be overwhelming. A committee might be inclined to weigh social burdens too heavily, particularly burdens on the resources of the committee's hospital or institution. Thus, sparing infants a hopeless life of meaningless suffering should be the only justification for active euthanasia.

Morris's statement of the conditions in which active euthanasia would be appropriate is thus not acceptable. No short verbal formulation is likely to do more than indicate a general standard of when life for the child is pointless misery. Morris's proposal perhaps overemphasizes rationality; indeed, that seems to be its main criterion. It omits, or seems to omit, cases in which there is some rationality, but also a life of painful operations. A better standard is a variation of that formulated above, namely, the child will lack capacities and opportunities for enjoyable experiences and fulfilling interests and desires, and unpleasant experiences and unfulfilled interests (desires) will render life one of pointless suffering. The fundamental basis must be that continued life is a clear harm to the individual whose life it is.

Given these or similar modifications, legalization of active euthanasia for severely defective children is acceptable. Instances of its use should be

[19]See Robert P. Hudson, "Death, Dying, and the Zealous Phase," in *Medical Treatment of the Dying: Moral Issues,* ed. Michael D. Bayles and Dallas M. High (Cambridge, Mass.: G. K. Hall & Company and Schenkman Publishing Company, 1978), pp. 65–84.

quite rare. Usually, passive euthanasia is preferable. Active euthanasia can be rationally appropriate only for the most extreme and rare cases. Nonetheless, the rarity should not detract from the importance of preventing pointless, unmitigated suffering.

Allocation of Resources

A general policy issue has been mentioned at various points in this discussion—the cost of care of defective infants. It pertains at two different levels—individual families and society, especially in providing neonatal intensive care facilities. Because this policy issue is a background to several issues previously discussed, it requires separate discussion.

In Case 5.1, Charles and Darlene do not have enough money to pay for Bernice's medical care. Long-term care for her is simply beyond their financial capacity. For example, the hospital costs for one week of care for mother and child in a case like Bernice's when treatment is not provided would be over $5,000. Surgery on the back and placement of a shunt would be another $3,000. In 1979, the cost of care for a child with a neural tube defect was about $60,000 to state public health systems.[20] Even for a relatively well-off family, without health insurance the costs of caring for a child with significant defects can be overwhelming. These costs make the familial burdens very great, perhaps intolerable. Thus, since the burden to parents and others is an ethical reason for not treating, money becomes important. The simple fact is that whether parents are or are not wealthy can make a difference to whether children should be treated.

Many people say that money should not make a difference in treatment decisions; that valuable lives should be saved whatever the cost. After all, what is money compared to human life? This attitude is naive. It is not simply money that is at stake but the alternative uses to which the money can be put. Parents can foresee that spending money for special education for a severely retarded child might mean they cannot afford to send another child to college, even though the latter child might benefit more from the college education than the retarded child from special education. The issue is not money versus health care, it is health care versus other, perhaps equally important, goods for other people. People misstate the issue by defining it in terms of the good or service that can be bought on the one hand—health care—but not specifying the good or service that is the likely alternative for the expenditure of funds.

The financial burdens at the familial level are largely, but not entirely, an aspect of the policies for funding health care. In the United States, they are partly due to the lack of national health insurance. In Canada, where national health insurance exists, couples do not have to worry about the direct costs of basic health care for a seriously ill or defective infant. There are other expenses that they will incur, and these can be quite significant, but hospital and doctor bills are not among them. In the United States, Medicaid will pay for hospital and doctor expenses, if one becomes poor

[20]See William R. Barclay and others, "The Ethics of In Utero Surgery," *JAMA*, 246, no. 14 (Oct. 2, 1981), 1554.

enough. But a family must become nearly destitute before Medicaid becomes operable. In many states, crippled children's services or children's hospitals are available for parents who are not as destitute as Medicaid requires.

The important point is that since decisions about treating infants should not depend significantly on the relative wealth of parents, a government policy or program to ensure payment of the major expenses should exist. Whether infants should live or die, be treated or not, should not depend primarily on the wealth of their parents. To make such basic treatment decisions depend on these considerations is to deny infants fundamental equality of opportunity and consideration. It is especially anomalous for the U.S. federal government to try to mandate such treatment when the government is reducing funds for such care.[21]

Even if governmental programs provide for the costs of medical care for defective newborns, questions of the allocation of resources still arise, only now at the social level. In 1979, the total cost of state crippled children's services was $200 million, and that does not include private and federal expenditures.[22] A few years ago the funds that one state government had allocated for medical care of defective newborns of poor parents were spent in the first nine months of the year. The bulk of the allocation, almost a million dollars, was spent on about fifteen infants who received long-term intensive care. Most infants spend about two weeks in such care, but a few infants may be treated for months or even years. The treatment of one such infant for six months is the equivalent of treating thirteen average infants. Each neonatal intensive care bed costs about half a million dollars to purchase, plus operating costs of nurses and staff.

Probably the only way to limit social costs is to limit the availability of treatment facilities. With limited facilities, not all infants can be treated; some criteria of selection for treatment are needed. There are three basic types of policies available for selecting infants for treatment, although various mixes of them are possible. Available facilities can be allocated on a "first come, first served" basis. This ensures that the facilities are fully utilized and does not discriminate among patients on the basis of social value. The major difficulty is that the available facilities might become fully utilized by infants with very poor prospects. Later-born infants, who would have good prognoses if treated, would be denied access. Hence, perhaps none would survive when many could have.

A second type of policy tries to correct for this difficulty by removing infants from intensive care if other infants with better prognoses need the units. At a conference in 1975, a number of experts from various fields supported such a policy.[23] But there are several drawbacks. First, it would be unusually cruel to parents to start their child on treatment and then cease to provide it because a child with better prospects came along. One might respond that only dying children would be removed from units. But if infants are dying, then it is probably best to remove them from useless treat-

[21]See Fost, "Putting Hospitals on Notice," p. 7.

[22]Barclay, "The Ethics of In Utero Surgery," p. 1554.

[23]Albert R. Jonsen and Michael J. Garland, eds., *Ethics of Newborn Intensive Care* (Berkeley, Calif.: Institute of Governmental Studies, 1976), p. 191.

ments, whether or not other infants need the unit. In addition, such a policy would involve physicians in making cost/benefit judgments about patients. They would have to decide whether it would be more useful to expend resources on one patient, or on another. Such activities would be destructive of the physician/patient/parent relationship. Finally, candidates for a neonatal intensive care unit would come from different physicians, who might, in order to get their patients admitted, be encouraged to portray their prospects as better than they are. In short, it would probably promote competition among physicians in getting patients admitted for care.

The third type of policy is to specify by condition certain classes of patients who will not be treated. Paul Ramsey favors such a policy, which he calls one of "medical indications."[24] He believes that such a policy is the only one that acknowledges the equal and independent value of lives.[25] Ramsey generally opposes using different standards for letting normal or defective children die; that is, he is opposed to making decisions based on judgments of the expectable value of life to the infants, which he calls "quality of life considerations."[26] However, almost any categories of illness or defect used for a medical indications policy will ultimately rest on quality or value of life considerations. For example, suppose one did not admit infants with myelomeningocele above the lumbar region. The reason for using such a medical classification would be the prognostic outcome in terms of longevity, paralysis, mental retardation, and so forth.

An example of such a possible policy can be based on a study of hospital costs for infants in an intensive care unit.[27] The study was based on charges during 1976–78, and the amounts would have to be increased to account for inflation since then. Three medical factors were found to best account for costs—low birth weight, need for surgery, and need for ventilation for more than twenty-four hours. Infants with all three factors constituted less than 3 percent of admissions but more than 9 percent of the total costs for treating all infants in the study, whereas infants with none of the factors constituted almost half the admissions but accounted for only 10 percent of total costs.[28] One may also plausibly assume that infants with all three factors had among the poorest mortality and morbidity outcomes. And high mortality serves to decrease costs. Thus, they might be a prime group not to be admitted.

Thus, to control social costs, the availability of treatment facilities should be limited. With limited facilities, one should then adopt a policy of selective admissions excluding infants with certain categories of defects or conditions. The reasons for such categories would often be the expectable value of life to infants if treated, but not all such decisions need be for such reasons. One excluding infants of less than 800 grams (1 lb. 12 oz.) and

[24]Ramsey, *Ethics at the Edges of Life,* p. 264.

[25]*Ibid.,* p. 262.

[26]*Ibid.,* p. 192.

[27]Ciaran S. Phibbs, Ronald L. Williams, and Roderic H. Phibbs, "Newborn Risk Factors and Costs of Neonatal Intensive Care," *Pediatrics,* 68, no. 3 (1981), 313–21.

[28]*Ibid.,* p. 320.

twenty-four weeks gestational age might relate simply to prospects for survival, if surviving infants of that weight and age have the same rate of defects as those of 1500 grams (3 lbs. 5 oz.) but fewer of them survive. Of course, the criteria used would have to change as medical technology improved and infants who previously had poor prospects came to have good ones. This change, however, should be based on clear evidence.

One final policy question remains. As an extreme possibility in allocating resources, Ramsey suggests redirecting money from pediatrics and neonatal intensive care to public health and preventive care.[29] He seems to think such a proposal fantastical, and perhaps it is, if it means shutting down all neonatal intensive care facilities. However, if one's goal is to reduce the number of seriously ill and defective infants born, and to increase the value of life to those who live, a significant shift in the current ratio of resources is not fantastic. Indeed, there are good reasons for such a policy.

Many untoward outcomes in childbirth are due to inadequate prenatal care, poor nutrition, and general poverty. These factors account for many premature and low birth-weight infants, who constitute a large proportion of infants in neonatal intensive care units. Genetic factors are not determined by such conditions, but many defective infants can be detected by prenatal diagnosis and aborted or treated so as to minimize handicaps. Bernice might not have been born with her defects if better prenatal care had been available; prenatal screening could have detected the defect. However, women like Darlene often cannot afford to see a physician for prenatal care during much of pregnancy. In North America, money has been disproportionately allocated to high technology intensive care over preventive measures. A better balance between the two is needed. More expenditures on prevention would decrease the births of infants with defects, would mean that more infants carried to term would have prospects for normal and valuable lives, and would decrease the need for intensive care units. Current policy emphasizes repairing defects after they occur rather than preventing them in the first place. It is an irrational allocation of resources, because it does not use the most effective means for attaining normal infants with prospects for lives found valuable. It is also inhumane. Many infants born premature and ill could have been born healthy had their mothers had adequate care.

BIBLIOGRAPHY

Duff, Raymond S. "Counseling Families and Deciding Care of Severely Defective Children: A Way of Coping with 'Medical Vietnam'," *Pediatrics,* 67, no. 3 (1981), 315–20.

Fost, Norman "Counseling Families Who Have a Child with a Severe Congenital Anomaly," *Pediatrics,* 67, no. 3 (1981), 321–324.

———— "Putting Hospitals on Notice," *The Hastings Center Report,* 12, no. 4 (August 1982), 5–8.

"Infants." *Encyclopedia of Bioethics,* (1978), 2, 717–51.

Jonsen, Albert R.; and Garland, Michael J., eds. *Ethics of Newborn Intensive Care.* Berkeley, Calif.: Institute of Governmental Studies, 1976.

[29]Ramsey, *Ethics at the Edges of Life,* p. 261–62.

KOHL, MARVIN, ed. *Infanticide and the Value of Life.* Buffalo, N.Y.: Prometheus Books, 1978.

STINSON, ROBERT; and STINSON, PEGGY "On the Death of a Baby," *Atlantic Monthly* (July 1979), 64–72.

SWINYARD, CHESTER A., ed. *Decision Making and the Defective Newborn: Proceedings of a Conference on Spina Bifida and Ethics.* Springfield, Ill.: Charles C. Thomas Publisher, 1978.

CHAPTER 6

The Future

Human reproduction has changed in remarkable ways during this century. Five main changes have already occurred or are likely to occur in the foreseeable future. First, couples can now have sexual intercourse without fear of conception. Possible future developments in this area are not likely to create ethical issues significantly different from those that have already arisen and been considered by society. Of the five basic changes, this is one of the two that have already become widely practiced.

The second major change is that reproduction can occur without sexual intercourse. Artificial insemination was the first aspect of this, and now *in vitro* fertilization has removed conception from the human body. These changes have not yet been adequately assimilated into the ethics of society. Nor do most people in society practice them, and it is doubtful that they ever will. In one possible futuristic scenario, most conceptions occur in laboratories, and couples then choose embryos on the basis of genetic characteristics of the expected child.

The third major change has been the development of abilities to predict accurately before birth the probability that a child will have certain genetic characteristics. The abilities are these: to separate sperm according to sex, significantly increasing the chances of a child of a particular sex; to detect that potential parents carry genes that may cause their offspring to have genetic defects; and to detect genetic and congenital defects in fetuses. So far, the ability to predict genetic characteristics has been confined to rather simple conditions, those based on single genes or for which simple markers can be detected, such as spina bifida. Genetic screening is becoming widely available and before long all pregnancies may be screened for a large number of characteristics besides Rh compatibility. Spina bifida can now be easily detected in almost all pregnancies. In the future, it may be possible to influence characteristics by intentionally introducing genes.

The fourth change, which is also widely practiced, is the improved ability to treat diseases and defects in newborn infants. As we saw in the last chapter, methods of treatment are still developing rapidly. Low birth-weight and premature infants now have much greater chances for normal survival than even a decade ago. Defects such as spina bifida can now also be treated more successfully than before, providing infants greater chances for a valuable life. Significant further gains in the ability to treat defects and diseases are on the immediate horizon.

The fifth change has not yet occurred. This is the ability to generate a viable human being completely outside the human body. *In vitro* fertilization permits genesis outside the body for a week or two. Developments in neonatology have made it possible for many neonates to survive outside the womb at twenty-four weeks gestation or even less. Consequently, it is only for the intervening period of about twenty to twenty-two weeks that fetuses cannot yet survive outside the womb. Whether artificial wombs will ever become a reality is unclear.

Future developments are most likely to pertain to the last three areas: genetic prediction, treatment, and ectogenesis (development outside the womb). One cannot accurately predict what developments will occur, let alone when. Some possible developments are now in the experimental stage. Others do not confront any known theoretical difficulties—only technical ones that could possibly be overcome with concentrated research. Because scientific developments cannot be predicted, the selection of issues in this chapter is somewhat arbitrary. The decisions have been based on what people have discussed, what seems possible in the near future, and what may raise significant moral issues. Some case studies (scenarios) are, of course, theoretical.

Cloning

Scenario 6.1 Francine is a brilliant microbiologist at State University. At the age of thirty-three she has already made major contributions to virology, discovering the viruses that cause several diseases and developing a cure for one of them. Because of her devotion to her career, Francine has not had time for many interpersonal relationships, and she has not found any male she wants to marry. Nonetheless, she would like to have a child. One of her colleagues has told her that society needs more people like her, who can make brilliant contributions to science. Thus, she decides to have herself cloned; the child will have exactly the same genetic makeup as Francine. To the extent that her abilities are genetically determined, the child will have the same ones. And Francine will assure that her daughter has the best available education.

Cloning has stirred the public's imagination and fears. It involves producing someone with the same genetic makeup as the donor-parent. To date, human beings have not been cloned. Mammals (mice) have been. At least two different processes for cloning are possible, but only one of them would reproduce an individual adult human. This process involves removing or destroying the nucleus of a fertilized egg and inserting the nucleus from a donor cell. The primary technical difficulty is finding a suitable donor cell. Although all cells in the human body contain the complete genetic code, this code is differentially switched on and off so that cells will form the different parts of the body. Consequently, in order to have a suitable nucleus for implanting, one must either find a cell that has not differentiated or be able to switch off the signals that made it specialize. So far, laboratory work has used the nuclei of cells at an early stage of differentiation. It is not clear whether cells from later stages of differentiation will work.

There are two basic types of reasons for the use of human cloning. One reason is the desire to have genetic offspring. Unlike reproduction using the genetic contribution from two people, cloning implies that the offspring will be genetically identical to the genetic parent. Thus, Francine's child would be genetically identical to her, as an identical twin would be. The difference is that in Francine's scenario, her clone would be thirty-three or so years younger. The second reason for cloning is to reproduce people with special talents, like Francine, for the benefit of society.

In Chapter 1, it was argued that a desire to beget genetic offspring is irrational. Essentially, two reasons supported that conclusion: namely, that little rewarding experience is involved in being a mere genetic donor, and that genetic offspring would be quite different from the parent. The first reason still pertains to cloning. Francine, however, is also going to raise the child, so she will have the experience of rearing. Thus, to consider cloning versus other options available to her, such as artificial insemination by donor, one must focus on the difference between those methods of acquiring a child to rear. This focuses on the importance of genetic contribution.

Reasons for cloning based on the desire for genetic offspring and on social benefit both depend on the clone being like the parent. To the extent that clones vary from the donors, they more closely resemble offspring resulting from the genetic contributions of two persons, and the expectable social benefits are less assured. Evidence about the similarity of a clone and donor can come only from identical twins. Identical twins are distinct persons whose personalities do differ. Since Francine's child would be raised in a different social and home environment—thirty-odd years later—this will also have an impact on her development. Consequently, one cannot expect the clone to resemble Francine any more than identical twins raised in separate families resemble each other. How much her clone will resemble Francine in emotional and intellectual characteristics depends on the relative contributions of genetics and environment (learning).

One might expect some important differences and burdens on the clone. If Francine or others try to raise the clone to be like Francine, they may stifle the clone's individuality and originality. These are two of the most important characteristics in people who, like Francine, make major contributions to society. Attempts to make the clone like Francine will probably destroy the very characteristics that make Francine specially valuable to society. To the extent that one fosters individuality and originality in the clone, she becomes different from Francine. Thus, the very attempt to create a clone closely resembling a person of special abilities is likely to be self-defeating.

The psychological pressures on the clone-child could significantly disrupt her emotional and intellectual development. If Francine and others pressure her daughter to develop in certain ways, the demands could be quite disruptive. Many children now have serious psychological difficulties because their parents have tried to make them in some desired mold—musicians, ball players, and so forth. Even without psychological pressure from Francine and others, the child might learn of her genetic endowment and feel pressure to live up to her mother's achievements. This constant unstated pressure can be quite damaging to children. It would be especially harmful if, due to environmental and learning situations, the daughter did not have the emotional or psychological inclinations to succeed in those respects.

The differences between a clone and donor are likely to be great enough to undercut reasons based on social benefit and desire for genetic offspring. In short, there is little reason to expect sufficient similarities in the important respects to justify cloning over artificial insemination from a carefully screened donor, and the possibilities of harmful effects on the clone-child make it inadvisable. If the object is to increase human talent, one would be better advised to develop the unused talent which already exists. Cloning of human beings is not desirable.

One possible variation on cloning involves different considerations. It might be possible to clone individuals in a somewhat different way and then take organs from developing embryos and culture them. In this way, bone marrow, kidneys, hearts, and other organs could be developed for transplantation without problems of rejection. Some organ-culturing is currently possible with mice and rats.

Two ethical concerns with this procedure can be mentioned. First, some people would have significant concerns about the destruction of embryos used to start the organ culture. As was argued in Chapter 3, such early stage embryos or fetuses lack moral status. Thus, this concern is not sound. Second, one might doubt that this sort of effort to keep people alive should be made. Perhaps people should accept their finitude and mortality. This question, and the whole topic of organ culture, is beyond the scope of this book.

Embryo-Fetal Engineering

Developments in genetics and *in vitro* fertilization open possibilities of modifying genetic characteristics of embryos. This discussion focuses on early stage embryos, well before they achieve moral status. The concern here is with engineering such beings into existence. Essentially, three types of genetic engineering are possible. First, embryos produced by *in vitro* fertilization might be screened for genetic defects prior to implantation. Second, embryos might be genetically modified to correct defects or introduce beneficial genetic features. Third, embryos consisting of cells with different genetic origins might be produced.

Embryo Screening

If conception occurs in the laboratory, it might be possible to screen embryos for genetic characteristics. An early suggestion of Dr. Robert Edwards, who with Dr. Patrick Steptoe developed the first successful "test tube" baby, was that *in vitro* fertilization might permit screening of embryos for sex.[1] Other characteristics, especially defects, might also be determined in the embryo stage.

To date, little success has been achieved in such screening. Some clinicians screen embryos by not implanting those that are slow in developing and thus might have genetic defects, but little else has yet been developed. Sex identification is so far not possible until about the time of implantation, too late to be of use. In the near future, various tests might be developed to determine whether an embryo has certain genetic defects; chromosomal defects such as Down syndrome probably will be among the first to be determined.

Screening embryos does not raise any issues we have not considered previously. Sex preselection has been discussed. The wrongness of its use for mere sexual preference does not depend on the method, so it is as unethical to separate embryos for this reason as it is to separate sperm. Screening embryos for genetic defects (including sex-linked defects) is generally the same as prenatal diagnosis, and would be preferable. It would avoid the risks of second-term abortions and the psychological costs of carrying a fetus only to lose it via induced or spontaneous abortion.

One concern about screening embryos is somewhat different, although it is similar to that about the use of *in vitro* fertilization: namely, the safety of the process. Chemical or microscopic examination of embryos could create defects. The very process of screening for one defect could introduce another one. Although embryos are rather resistant to damage and spontaneous abortions eliminate many serious defects, the central assurance of safety is adequate experimentation with animals prior to trials with human embryos. Even if the defects being screened do not occur in animals, animal embryos can be subjected to the same procedures, and the resulting animals checked for created defects. In the end, of course, one must simply determine whether the possible benefits of avoiding a defect by screening outweigh the risks of introducing other defects. At this time, it is difficult to determine whether that will be so.

Perhaps the best method of avoiding defects is to screen the donors of eggs and sperm. If parents are at significant risk of a genetic defect, then the principle concerning risk to the unborn implies that they should not reproduce. The only reason for not using donor sperm or eggs is the desire for genetic offspring. That desire, which is irrational, carries no weight against the principle of avoiding risk to the unborn.

Genetic Modification

Genetic modification can be used on an embryo or a fetus, either to correct a defect or to introduce some desired genetic feature. Such procedures can also be attempted on adults, and one unsuccessful attempt has

[1]Robert G. Edwards and David J. Sharpe, "Social Values and Research in Human Embryology," in *Selected Readings: Genetic Engineering and Bioethics,* ed. Robert A. Paoletti (New York: MSS Information Corporation, 1972), pp. 87–88.

already been made. The concern here is with such modification early in reproduction.

Scenario 6.2   Hilda is about ten weeks pregnant. She and her husband Glen are both carriers for sickle cell anemia. A new early test indicates that the fetus has the disease. Her doctor has suggested that she consider an experiment to correct the condition. The medical team would try to insert the correct blood gene into some cells of the fetus. If enough cells take up the gene, then enough of the fetus's blood cells will be normal to alleviate the effects of sickle cell disease. Of course, the child would still be likely to pass the gene on to its offspring; they would probably all be carriers at least.

The same type of procedure as in Scenario 6.2 could also be attempted on an embryo. This presumes the capacity to screen embryos for sickle cell disease. The chances of success with an embryo would be greater than with a fetus because fewer cells need to receive the new gene. It might be possible to affect the reproductive cells so that the trait would not be transmitted.

Besides trying to correct defects, similar procedures might be used to try to introduce desired genetic traits in embryos or fetuses without any known defect. Such procedures are at best in the far distant future. Most human characteristics that are valued—intelligence, friendliness, and so forth—are either dependent on multiple genes or perhaps on environmental nurture. So undoubtedly, in terms of technical feasibility and desirability, the case would be stronger for correcting genetic defects.

It is not acceptable to attempt such early genetic modification, even to correct defects. Compared to the alternatives, such modification is not worth trying. If a defect is discovered in an embryo, an alternative to attempting modification is simply not to implant it. Attempts at modification might or might not be successful, and might risk introducing other defects. Destruction of the embryo and creation of another for implantation is preferable. The choice is between a risk of significant defect with this embryo and use of another embryo without such a risk. Because embryos do not have moral status, the principle concerning risk to the unborn indicates that such attempts at genetic modification are ethically wrong.

Essentially the same argument applies to attempts at modifying defects in fetuses before they have the moral status of a right to life. Either the defect is sufficiently serious to justify abortion followed by a new pregnancy, as in the case of Hilda, or it is not sufficiently serious to risk the modification. One might dispute whether a fetus with sickle cell disease should be aborted, but if it should not be, that is because one believes that the child's life would not be very seriously affected. Alternatively, suppose the fetus had galactosemia, which can be effectively handled by eliminating milk and milk products from the child's diet. Although this requires considerable care, the child can live a relatively normal life. One should not risk the introduction of other genetic defects, perhaps quite serious, in order to attempt to cure the fetus so that it can later consume milk and milk products.

If genetic modification of embryos and fetuses is not justifiable to correct defects, then it is not justifiable to try to introduce desired characteristics. One would be risking the introduction of defects into an essentially normal embryo or fetus in the hopes of producing some desired characteristic. The chances of harm and benefit might be about equal, so there is no net gain. The principle regarding risk to the unborn again applies. If one wants to provide the child with better abilities, one can provide advantages after it is born, such as better education and so forth. These methods are much less likely to harm, and more likely to benefit, than genetic modification. Even if genetic traits were introduced, most would require such a favorable environment for their expression.

Chimeras

The type of engineering involved here overlaps somewhat with the forms of modification just discussed. In genetic modification, specific genes are introduced. That could be involved here, but the difference is that the genes would come from a different species. In effect, there are two forms of chimera production as meant here. One form is the introduction of genes of one species into another. This can involve introducing nonhuman genes into human embryo cells or human genes into nonhuman embryos. The other form is to mix cells of different embryos.

So far, the only actual practice has been to mix embryo cells from two different strains of the same species—mice. For example, one can take cells from embryos of two differently colored strains of mice and mix them together in one embryo. The result is a mouse with splotches of each color.

People are apt to become quite upset at the thought of introducing human genes into nonhuman species. Indeed, this has resulted in some philosophical discussion about how human beings with moral status could be distinguished from other animals.[2] One must consider carefully what human genetic material is. The genetic code of all cells consists of strands of a few basic chemicals in different series. When one speaks of introducing human genes, what one means is introducing sequences of these chemicals found only in humans. Many of the sequences found in human beings are also found in other species. Consequently, in introducing genetic elements, one need not be introducing anything recognizably human as most people think of humans, for example, a face or head. One is introducing chemicals already found in the other species, but not in that particular sequence. Of course, one might introduce larger blocks of human genetic information, such as a whole chromosome.

What would be the point of such manipulations? In animal husbandry, there might be considerable advantage from modifying species, such as cattle, to yield more meat and so forth. For example, one such genetic combination that has been performed, although not in a laboratory, is to cross the North American bison with a form of cattle, to produce a beefalo. The point was to produce more meat than buffalo do, and a hardier breed than cattle. It is unlikely that human genetic characteristics would be valuable for such purposes.

Perhaps a technically easier development, but a rather unlikely one, is to mix cells from two human embryos, or cells of some other species and a

---

[2]See, for example, Paul Ramsey, *Fabricated Man: The Ethics of Genetic Control* (New Haven and London: Yale University Press, 1970), pp. 81–86.

human embryo.[3] Again, one must ask what the purpose of such a mixture would be. The purpose of correcting defects is subject to the same arguments as against genetic modification. No other plausible purpose has yet been suggested. One farfetched suggestion has been to make short people, or perhaps people with no legs, for space flights.

There are two major objections to such genetic engineering with human beings. First, any results different enough to be worth striving for would constitute some type of "freak." This term is used advisedly, because those beings would likely be subject to the sorts of discrimination and negative attitudes that the word suggests. Assuming that these beings would be intelligent and sensitive, they would be subjected to severe psychological distress in human interactions. With the principle regarding risk to the unborn, this reason in itself is sufficient to make it wrong to produce them.

Second, it is unlikely that such beings would serve any plausible purpose. Any tasks that they might perform better than average human beings can probably be performed, and performed better, by machines. Most of the work of flying space ships and the space shuttle is done by computers directing machinery. They are faster in making decisions, capable of taking more factors into account, and more reliable.

At least at this point, no reason exists to create such human chimeras. Their development would cause the chimeras themselves much suffering, and would be wrong. Perhaps animal chimeras would be useful for producing food or for other purposes, but not any sufficiently human to be recognizable as such—having human physical features or intelligence.

In Utero Treatment

Case 6.3 Ida is twenty-one weeks pregnant. She has undergone prenatal diagnosis which shows that her fetus has hydrocephalus (water on the brain). The doctors explain to her and her husband, Jesse, that progressive increase of the fluid in the fetus's brain will greatly enlarge its head, probably causing mental retardation. However a new method of treatment permits the insertion of a shunt into the fetus's head to drain off the excess fluid and allow nearly normal development. The procedure is not guaranteed to work. There is an increased risk of premature labor or spontaneous abortion. The risk to Ida is rather small; a local anesthetic would be used and a needle inserted into the uterus as in fetoscopy. The alternatives are to abort, or to continue the pregnancy without treatment and with a greater risk of mental retardation or more severe retardation.

Ida and Jesse discuss these alternatives. They would really like to have another child, and neither approves of abortion unless there is practically no chance that the fetus will have a meaningful life. In the end, they decide to let the doctors implant the shunt.

---

[3]One does mix cells from two different humans in bone marrow transplants and by introducing cells to produce enzymes and correct for inborn errors of metabolism. In these cases, however, one is usually dealing with people with the moral status of a right to life.

The procedure offered to Ida and Jesse is only one of a large number of new techniques for treating the fetus to improve outcomes.[4] For some conditions, early labor can be induced so that the fetus can be treated outside the womb. In other cases, such as myelomeningocele, the fetus can be delivered by cesarean section, which carries a lower risk that membranes will be ruptured and become infected than does a vaginal delivery. For other problems, medication can be given, either to the pregnant woman or to the fetus itself through the amniotic fluid. Finally, as in this case, surgery can be performed on the fetus. Such a technique has been used for some time to change completely the blood in the fetus for Rh incompatibility. Besides the surgery in Case 6.3, surgery might be used to remove obstructions preventing the discharge of urine. This involves surgically opening the uterus and partly removing the fetus to operate on it. Surgery to close a spinal lesion is also possible.

Ethical Analysis

These techniques, some of which are currently available and others of which are in advanced experimental stages, complicate ethical and policy considerations but do not require new principles. Three primary ethical principles are involved. One is the principle regarding risk to the unborn. If the pregnancy is to continue to term, the treatments may decrease the chances of the child having a significant defect. Second, as we saw in Chapter 3, prior to twenty-eight weeks the fetus does not have a moral status sufficient to ground a right to life. Third, all these treatments involve doing something to the pregnant woman's body, so her right to control her body is involved. However, these three considerations are not affected to the same degree by the different forms of treatment.

The techniques of early labor and cesarean delivery do not create a significant ethical dilemma. These interventions are not likely to be medically plausible until the fetus has a right to life. The effects on the woman's body are not major. She will have to undergo delivery at some time. Having a cesarean delivery rather than a vaginal one is a more significant intrusion because the risks to her are greater. Nonetheless, when there is a significant chance of benefit to the fetus, the principle regarding risk to the unborn outweighs the risk to the woman and the treatment is ethically required. However, this is true only when the treatment has been proven to be of significant benefit.

The various treatments by medication are not much more difficult. In these cases, although the pregnant woman does not have to undergo the treatment or some comparable effect on her body no matter what, the risks to her from the medications are likely to be quite minimal. The risk to the woman from inserting medication into the amniotic fluid is not very great either. However, the risk to the fetus is somewhat greater, since premature delivery could be brought on, or, rarely, the fetus could be punctured. Consequently, if the fetus has a right to life and the treatment has been

[4]See Michael Harrison, Mitchell S. Golbus, and Roy A. Filly, "Management of the Fetus with a Correctable Congenital Defect," *JAMA,* 246, no. 7 (1981), 774–77.

shown to be substantially effective, then such treatment is ethically obligatory. If the fetus has not developed to the point of having a right to life, then abortion remains an option. Treatment is ethically appropriate only if the woman decides to carry to term.

The surgery option is not likely to arise when the fetus has a right to life; at that stage early delivery followed by surgery is probably medically preferable. However, it may arise occasionally. In such a situation, if the defect, even with treatment, would provide a life of such low quality that abortion for fetal defect would be justifiable, then that remains an option. But practically, an aborted fetus of that age is likely to live, so an abortion will have the same effect as early delivery.

The significant cases arise when the fetus has no right to life. If the child would have a significant handicap even with treatment, then the principle regarding risk to the unborn implies that abortion is appropriate. If the treatment can completely repair the problem, then the principle regarding risk to the unborn prohibits continuation of the pregnancy without treatment. Unfortunately, such cases are likely to be rare. For example, placing a shunt for hydrocephalus still requires another shunt after birth, and is not a guarantee of normal intelligence. Moreover, most defects open to surgical repair have other associated abnormalities. Nonetheless, the possibility of effective surgical treatment can change some cases from those in which the principle regarding risk to the unborn implies that abortion is an obligation, to those in which it is not.

Suppose, however, that the defect is not one that, untreated, would make abortion ethically obligatory. The less serious the defect, the smaller the benefit that can result from surgery. This makes it less likely that the benefits will outweigh the risks. Moreover, the risks include not only those of the fetus but also those of the pregnant woman. Surgery that involves opening the uterus poses a significantly greater risk to the woman than that involving insertion of a needle. Thus, usually such surgery is not ethically required. However, a pregnant woman can voluntarily assume risks to herself in order to continue the pregnancy and improve the chances that the child will be normal.

Finally, one must consider who should make the decision. In one center doing experimental surgery for hydrocephalus, people are appointed to serve as advocates for the fetus, although the final decision is left to the pregnant woman.[5] Such a procedure might serve some useful purpose; but, as the fetus has no right to life at this time, these advocates cannot ethically argue for the continuation of the pregnancy. Ethically, they can only represent the interests of the fetus should the woman decide to continue the pregnancy.

The decision-maker principle that a good reason for persons making decisions is that they will bear most of the consequences applies here. It implies that the pregnant woman should make the decision. First, abortion is an option, and we have seen that women alone should decide about abortion. Second, unlike decisions about defective newborns, the woman here is directly affected—she is also a patient of the surgery. One might

[5]William H. Clewell and others, "A Surgical Approach to the Treatment of Fetal Hydrocephalus," *New England J. Med.*, 306, no. 22 (1982), 1325.

claim that this implies that she has a greater conflict of interest than in decisions about defective newborns and so should not make the decision. However, the burden of surgery is not likely to be greater than the burden involved in care of a defective newborn. Moreover, her right to control her body is involved. Although the father should not have control over a decision whether to abort, normally he ethically should be consulted by the woman as to whether to have the surgery if she does not abort.

Policy Analysis

The major policy question is whether a woman's decision against treatment could ever be overridden by a court. Obviously, as long as abortion is legally permissible, a court cannot override a decision to have an abortion. If the woman decides against abortion, or the fetus has a right to life, then surgery might be required. However, such cases are likely to be few. The considerations that apply are the same as those developed in Chapter 4 for court-ordered cesarean delivery. First, the treatment would have to be established. No court should have the power to order someone to undergo medical experimentation. Second, the potential benefits would have to outweigh the risks (including those to the woman) significantly. Because the woman's right to control her body is being invaded, the benefit to the fetus must be great enough to outweigh both the risks and the woman's right. Third, the court must have clear and convincing evidence that the surgery will be beneficial. The underlying rationale is that the woman is not justified in taking a risk with the fetus's health that would amount to child neglect or abuse if the child was already alive.

A court is more likely to be able justifiably to require a woman to undergo the other forms of treatment. First, the fetus will probably have a right to life. Second, the risks to the woman, and thus the invasion of her right to control her body, are likely to be less. As we saw in Chapter 4, a court can be justified in ordering a cesarean delivery, and the same applies to medication.

Ectogenesis

The last topic is developing an artificial placenta or womb so that the full development of a human embryo-fetus can occur outside of another human being. Such a possibility recalls images from Aldous Huxley's *Brave New World* of human infants being "decanted" from their test tubes.

Such a technology could have several purposes. One would be to permit better scientific study of fetal development in the hope that the causes of congenital defects can be discovered and cured or prevented. Another possible purpose is to avoid risks to the fetus from the rather uncontrolled environment of the womb. The fetal environment could be carefully monitored and controlled under laboratory conditions to avoid risks. Another purpose would be so that a woman without a uterus could have a child. Yet another, which is really partial ectogenesis, would be to save spontaneously aborted fetuses. A final purpose would be to make surgery and other treatment easier.

Considering these purposes or reasons in reverse order, the last one does not appear persuasive. Proportionately few fetuses require treatment, and these cannot be detected in advance. (If they could be, it would be wrong to gestate them.) Even fewer are amendable to treatment. Consequently, at most, one out of a hundred could be helped. With abortion as a viable alternative, there is no reason to use ectogenesis for all or most fetuses in order to help a very few.

Nor does the purpose of saving spontaneously aborted fetuses justify ectogenesis. Few spontaneous abortions occur in or near a hospital, so the chances of getting a fetus to an artificial womb in time to have any significant chance of normal survival is minimal. The possible success does not seem to justify the risk, especially when another pregnancy is possible and such a high percentage of spontaneously aborted fetuses are abnormal.

Neither is the purpose of allowing women who lack uteruses to have children persuasive. *In vitro* fertilization and a surrogate mother can accomplish the same end. Apparently, implantation can occur generally in the abdominal cavity, although not yet with normal fetal development, so surgical reconstruction of the uterus might be possible. This would enable the woman to have the experience of bearing a child. It might be suggested that the idea is to enable women to avoid having to bear a child. Their careers, health, and so forth would not be affected. However, *in vitro* fertilization with her ova and a uterine mother would again accomplish the same end.

One purpose of ectogenesis could be to avoid the very real risks to the fetus involved in gestation and delivery. The risks of use of an artificial womb must be placed in opposition to this. Adjusting nutrients, chemical balances, and so forth in a laboratory probably carries risks of mistake as high as the risks in nature. It is quite a different matter to use an incubator to save the life of a very premature infant than it is deliberately to set out to use an artificial womb when no life with moral status exists. At present it is unclear to what extent the variability among humans is due, if at all, to differences in experience in the womb. Artificial wombs would remove these differences. They might produce children with less variability. Some people might find that attractive, but others would find the loss of human variability a detraction from life. Much would depend on the amount of sameness that resulted. It is doubtful that a uniform fetal environment would eliminate a great deal of human variability, which is probably more due to differences in genetic inheritance and childhood experiences. Consequently, this consideration is not a positive reason for ectogenesis. If one has considerable faith in the ability of science and technology to produce a reliable artificial womb it might be an acceptable use.

The purpose of permitting better scientific understanding of fetal development and the causes of defects and disease cannot provide a reason for the widespread use of ectogenesis. At best, this supports its use in scientific studies, not for general human reproduction. Much might be learned by experiments with fetuses in artificial wombs. It is not clear how much more could be learned by the technique versus tissue and organ culture, but it is likely that more could be learned concerning the relationships and interactions of various parts of the whole organism.

The ethics of such experimental use of ectogenesis depend on the status of fetuses. As we saw, fetuses do not have moral status for a right not to suffer needless pain until about the fourth month, and the seventh month for a right to life. Consequently, fetal experimentation is not wrong in itself. Of course, experiments can be unethical due to their purposes, or for reasons independent of being experiments on fetuses. Because experiments might introduce defects, any fetuses used for these purposes should not be brought to term. They could not be developed beyond the sixth month without creating beings with a right to life. Consequently, limited development of fetuses in artificial wombs for experimental purposes is acceptable, provided no pain is caused and they are not allowed to develop to a state of consciousness. Of course, these restrictions apply to setting out to develop a fetus in an artificial womb, not to experimental attempts to save very premature infants.

Overall, most of the beneficial aspects of new methods of human reproduction currently exist—artificial insemination, *in vitro* fertilization, genetic screening, and improving pregnancy outcome. One can expect improvements in these methods, particularly the ability to detect genetic and congenital defects at earlier stages of gestation and treatment to improve outcome.

The futuristic methods of human reproduction considered in this chapter are not generally ethically acceptable. Cloning is not likely to produce the benefits people think, and it is likely to result in psychological harm to the clones; other methods are available to increase the human talent available. While embryo screening is ethically preferable to screening at later stages of development, genetic modification and the production of chimeras would seriously risk harm to those persons produced, without offering discernible benefits. Similarly, ectogenesis does not offer likely human benefit in comparison with other alternatives—except for limited scientific purposes and raising very premature fetuses whose gestation began in a uterus.

BIBLIOGRAPHY

BARCLAY, WILLIAM R.; and others "The Ethics of In Utero Surgery," *Journal of the American Medical Association,* 246, no. 14 (1981), 1550–55.

GROBSTEIN, CLIFFORD *From Chance to Purpose: An Appraisal of External Human Fertilization.* Reading, Mass.: Addison-Wesley Publishing Company, Advanced Book Program, 1981. Chaps. 3, 6.

HARRISON, MICHAEL R.; GOLBUS, MITCHELL S.; and FILLY, ROY A. "Management of the Fetus With a Correctable Congenital Defect," *Journal of the American Medical Association,* 246, no. 7 (1981), 774–77.

Note, "Asexual Reproduction and Genetic Engineering: A Constitutional Assessment of the Technology of Cloning," 47 *Southern California Law Review* 476–584 (1974).

RAMSEY, PAUL *Fabricated Man: The Ethics of Genetic Control.* New Haven and London: Yale University Press, 1970. Chap. 2.

ROBERTSON, JOHN A. "The Right to Procreate and In Utero Fetal Therapy," *Journal of Legal Medicine,* 3, no. 3 (1982), 333–66.

RUDDICK, WILLIAM; and WILCOX, WILLIAM "Operating on the Fetus," *Hastings Center Report,* 12, no. 5 (Oct. 1982), 10–14.

Conclusion

In the course of examining the many aspects of human reproduction, we have discovered a few acceptable principles that provide guidance for most of the moral issues that arise. By way of conclusion, it is worth reviewing them and some of their uses. The principle of reproductive freedom is that people should not have parental responsibilities involuntarily, and people should have the opportunity to make a fully voluntary and informed choice to acquire them. It is justified primarily by the importance of people controlling their own lives, and the impact parenthood has on people's lives. This principle supports the availability of contraception, the consent of spouses to reproduction by AID and surrogate motherhood, and the permissibility of abortion for rape or incest, even if the fetus has a right to life.

Perhaps the most important principle is that concerning risk to the unborn; that it is wrong to take a substantial risk that an unborn child will have a significant defect or handicap. This principle is primarily supported by the facts that one would be responsible for the defect, and that it can be avoided without harm because the early fetus does not have moral status. This principle condemns would-be parents risking their child's well-being by conceiving when they have genetic or other risks of the fetus having a defect or disease; pregnant women from engaging in behaviors which risk damage to the fetus; women in high-risk pregnancies having homebirths; cloning; genetic modification; producing human chimeras; and failure to undergo *in utero* treatment for a fetus to be carried to term. The principle concerning risk to the unborn, with the principle of freedom of reproduction, supports genetic screening, including abortion of seriously affected fetuses prior to seven months.

The principle concerning the burdens to others was first formulated for decisions made when no being with moral status existed. In Chapter 5, we saw that it extends to issues about life-prolonging treatment for seriously defective or ill newborns. The extended principle is that the burden to others is a reason not to bring a child into existence or to prolong a child's existence. It is primarily a specification of the general principle that effects on all persons affected are relevant. This principle supports not conceiving children with defects, aborting fetuses with defects, and not providing life-prolonging treatment to seriously damaged or ill newborns (or fetuses) when it is debatable that their lives would be valuable to them.

The decision-maker principles are that good reasons for persons to make a decision are that they either have special relevant expertise or will bear most of the consequences. Although relevant to questions about childbirth, not treating defective newborns, and *in utero* treatment, the principle of expertise is not sufficient to justify physicians' making the major decisions on these matters, only acting as advisors. Instead, within limits based on the well-being of the child, pregnant women or parents should make these decisions because, next to the child, they bear most of the consequences. Parental decisions about childbirth were limited for high-risk pregnancies, and parental decisions concerning treatment of defective newborns or fetuses with a right to life were limited when life for infants would most likely be of significant benefit or harm to them.

Two other considerations were also important in many respects. First, a desire for genetic offspring is probably irrational, or at least not as important as often thought. This point plays a role in considering the morality of various new methods of conception, and of risking defects in a child. Second, fetuses lack moral status for a right not to suffer pain unnecessarily prior to four months and seven months for a right to life; prior to that, they lack the capacities for the types of experiences grounding such rights. This consideration is fundamental to the morality of abortion, and supports *in vitro* fertilization, embryo screening, and ectogenesis for scientific purposes.

In considering many aspects of human reproduction, it has been useful to consider alternatives. In Chapter 1, this meant considering how people can reproduce naturally. That single women could become pregnant by natural intercourse indicates that there is no special reason for or benefit from restricting artificial insemination or *in vitro* fertilization for single women. In looking at futuristic possibilities, it has been useful to consider whether they would bring any benefits not possible by existing techniques.

Despite all the modern scientific-technological means of reproduction, most people will probably continue to have children as they always have. The two basic rational desires in human reproduction are for a child to rear and for that child to be free of significant handicaps. Modern science has contributed to these ends. It has developed techniques, such as artificial insemination and *in vitro* fertilization, to enable people to have children to rear. It has also developed techniques to enable couples to avoid the conception or birth of infants with severe defects and to correct or alleviate many defects. These scientific advances have raised many of the moral issues we have examined. Partly due to these advances, much control of human reproduction, especially of the decisions about childbirth and defective newborns, has slipped from the hands of parents into the hands of physicians. This loss of control is not irreversible. Recently, the trend has reversed, in part due to the sensitive help of many physicians and other health care personnel.

On balance, human reproduction is better today than it has been, and with certain changes it can be a rewarding experience that has better chances than ever before of providing people with normal, wanted children—and only wanted children. In general, the ethically preferred future is one that improves on these changes with more sensitive childbirth and greater ability to screen for and treat defects, rather than one that for no rational purpose pursues cloning, genetic engineering, and production of chimeras. The goal is the reproduction of normal, wanted human beings to live in a decent society.

Cases and Scenarios
for Further Study

Cases

1. Alice goes to an infertility clinic. She tells the doctor that four years ago, when she was twenty-five years old, she was sterilized because she had had two children and she and her husband did not want any more. A year later they divorced. Now she has married Bill and would like to have his child. Consequently, she would like to have her sterilization reversed. Is it ethical for the physician to operate on Alice to try to open her tubes so that she can have another child? Why or why not? If that does not work, should the physician attempt *in vitro* fertilization? Why or why not? Should women who have never had children be given priority over Alice for IVF? Should government or private health insurance pay for Alice's treatment? The cost of IVF is about $20,000 for each child born.

2. Cloris and Dave had been unable to have children because Dave is sterile. They decide to use AID to have a child. Without telling Cloris, Dave asks the physician to use sperm from his married brother Edgar. The doctor agrees, but no one ever tells Cloris or Edgar's wife. Should semen from Edgar have been used? Was it ethical not to tell Cloris or Edgar's wife? Should there be a policy forbidding doctors to use sperm from close relatives of infertile husbands?

3. Florence goes to see Dr. Gregory at an infertility clinic. She explains that she is a lesbian living with another woman and that she very much wants to have a baby. Consequently, she wants AID. After reflection, Dr. Gregory artificially inseminates her with his own sperm. Should Dr. Gregory have inseminated her? Should he have used his own sperm?

4. Harriet and Ian already have a young child. They also want another one and think it would provide companionship for the one they presently have. Unfortunately, Ian has just started a fifteen-year prison sentence for armed robbery and conjugal visits are not allowed. Consequently, they

would like to have Harriet artificially inseminated with Ian's sperm (AIH). Should prison officials allow Ian to send his semen out of the prison?

5. Janice and Kevin have not been able to have a baby. The doctors cannot determine the cause. Finally, they try IVF. Janice takes drugs to produce extra eggs. One is placed in a dish with sperm from a donor to test whether there is some undetectable problem with Kevin's sperm. Kevin's sperm fail to fertilize an egg, but the donor's sperm do so. The doctors ask whether Janice and Kevin want to transfer the embryo fertilized by the donor. Would it be unethical for Janice and Kevin to use it?

6. After examining Louise, the doctors at an IVF clinic tell her that they cannot retrieve ova from her because of all the damage to her ovaries. She and Marty, her husband, will never be able to have a child who is genetically theirs. However, the clinic has a frozen embryo of a couple who had twins and do not wany any more children. This couple has given permission to transfer the embryo to another couple. Would it be unethical for Louise and Marty to agree to have the embryo transferred to Louise?

7. Nadine has just given birth to a baby boy after years of infertility. Unfortunately, the baby has many defects which do not correspond to any definite disease or condition. Moreover, Nadine was artificially inseminated with sperm from her husband Oswald as well as that from two donors. Thus, it is impossible to determine whether the baby's defects are due to a genetic condition of Nadine, Oswald, or a donor; to drug treatments Nadine and Oswald had; or to some other factor. What should Nadine and Oswald be told? Should sperm from the two donors no longer be used? What should Oswald's ethical and legal responsibilities be toward the baby?

8. Polly's and Queenie's brother died of Duchenne's muscular dystrophy. There is some possibility that they are carriers and that their sons might be affected. They were originally told that the chances that a son would have this defect were small. However, subsequent analysis of the family history indicates that the risk is about 2.5 percent. Queenie recently gave birth to a normal boy. Polly is now pregnant, but is opposed to abortion and probably would not have one even if she carried an affected son. Should she be contacted to determine whether she is a carrier and to offer amniocentesis?

9. Roslyn is thirty-nine years old and pregnant from IVF. The physicians offer her amniocentesis because of the increased risk of genetic abnormalities for a woman of her age, and the as yet unknown risk of defects due to IVF. However, there is a one-half to one percent chance of spontaneous abortion as a result of amniocentesis. Consequently, Roslyn refuses amniocentesis; she does not want to risk losing her baby, since this is probably her only chance to have a child. Is her decision ethically wrong? Should amniocentesis be required of all women undergoing IVF?

10. Sheila is an unmarried seventeen-year-old woman who lives with her mother. She is about twenty-seven to twenty-eight weeks pregnant and has complained that the fetus is not kicking much. An ultrasound examination reveals that the infant has a spina bifida lesion around the middle of the spinal column. It is not possible to determine the extent of the lesion and damage.

Three possible options are as follows: (1) Sheila could be informed, and an abortion could be performend if she so desired. However, abortions at this stage of pregnancy are legal only for the physical or mental health of the woman, not for fetal defect. An abortion at this point would have to be by hysterotomy, with the probability of a live birth. Premature "delivery" might cause signficant stress for the infant and would compound problems. (2) Sheila could be informed that it is likely that her infant has a defect but that it is impossible to tell exactly what the extent of the defect is. Sheila has completed only two years of high school, so it is not clear that she can completely grasp the significance of this information. Moreover, the anxiety caused by such information might adversely affect the pregnancy. (3) Information could be withheld from Sheila and arrangements made for immediate care of the infant on delivery. This would involve arranging for delivery in a hospital with neonatal intensive care facilities. What should the physician do?

11. Thelma is a twenty-five-year-old woman in an institution for mentally retarded persons. Her IQ is estimated to be 39, and she engages in psychotic behavior. She has previously been in two other institutions. Her father is seriously ill, and her mother has raised seven other children—six younger and one older. Thelma is found to be about four-and-a-half months pregnant. However, she is in good physical condition and the pregnancy appears normal. Nobody knows who the father is. Should Thelma have an abortion? Who should make the decision—Thelma, her parents, or the physicians at the institution?

12. Una is a twenty-two-year-old model. She has been living with Vincent for eight months. She is about a month-and-a-half pregnant. She was not very careful in taking her birth control pills. When she told Vincent she was pregnant, he seemed happy and wanted to get married. However, Una does not want to interrupt her career at this point. She has just received a couple of assignments from prominent firms. She loves Vincent and would like to marry him, but she does not want to have a baby now. Would it be unethical for Una to have an abortion?

13. Winnie, a fourteen-year-old, is very tearful when Dr. Xuan tells her that she is pregnant. Dr. Xuan asks her who the father is. At first Winnie refuses to tell. She insists that she does not have any boy friends. Finally, she admits that her father comes to bed with her when her mother is working nights. Dr. Xuan believes that Winnie is physically capable of carrying the fetus to term. However, there is an increased risk of genetic defect due to the incest, and the pregnancy is likely to be psychologically traumatic for Winnie. Is it ethical for Winnie to have an abortion?

14. This is Yvonne's first delivery. She and Zachary are both very excited by the time they reach the hospital. They have been to childbirth classes, and are looking forward to practicing all they have learned about natural childbirth. Dr. Abrams has been very cooperative, saying that he will go along with any reasonable request. The labor goes very well. When Yvonne goes to the delivery room, Zachary is delayed for a few minutes. When he arrives, Yvonne is crying. As Zachary tries to console her, she blurts out that Dr. Abrams gave her anesthesia. Zachary is mad and yells at Dr. Abrams, "Why? Why did you give her anesthetic? You know we did not want any unless it was necessary." Dr. Abrams looks up from having just completed an episiotomy and says, "Either you calm down or you will have to leave. I gave her an anesthetic because I thought it was necessary. You don't want me to take chances with your wife or baby do you?" The

delivery then goes well. From this information, do you think Dr. Abrams's conduct was unethical? Should Yvonne be entitled to sue him? If so, what sort of damages should she be entitled to? If not, why not?

15. Belinda and Caroline are both nurse-midwives. They have practiced with a physician for two years. Now they think they are ready to practice on their own. The physician they have been working with agrees to provide medical backup. They remortgage their houses and borrow more money to get the $50,000 needed to set up their clinic. Several women have already signed up for delivery, and Belinda and Caroline have only to get permission from the local hospital to do deliveries there. Much to their surprise, at the hearing the hospital board has on their application, the chief of obstetrics opposes their application. Although they have a fine physician to serve as medical backup, the chief contends that the physician's office is ten minutes from the hospital. If Belinda and Caroline had difficulties, the baby or mother could die before the physician could arrive. Moreover, they have not arranged for an alternative backup if the physician is out of town. Consequently, the chief contends, the risks are not acceptable. Moreover, should anything happen, the hospital might be found negligent and liable. Would it be unethical for the hospital board to refuse Belinda and Caroline permission to deliver at the hospital? What practical steps might be taken to overcome the objections of the chief of obstetrics?

16. Denise's baby boy is born at a nonhospital birthing center. During her pregnancy, there were no indications of complications. During delivery, everything appears to go smoothly, but at birth the infant has difficulty breathing. The doctor at the center calls for an ambulance to transport the baby to the nearest hospital, about twelve minutes away. However, the baby dies before it reaches the hospital. The evidence indicates that had it been put on a ventilator immediately, it probably would have lived. Was it ethically wrong for Denise to deliver at the birthing center when her baby would have lived had she delivered at the hospital? Why or why not?

17. Evita is twenty-six years old and lives with her current boyfriend, Felix, who works as a parking lot attendant. She is several months pregnant. When she visits a doctor, he notes that she appears to have a hangover. He explains to her that excessive drinking of alcohol during pregnancy might damage her baby. Evita tells him that she would never do anything to harm her baby. But, she continues, surely she should be able to have some fun now and then. The doctor says, "Sure, but just go easy on the alcohol." When she gets home, Evita tells Felix that the doctor was terrible, that he did not want her to do anything to have fun, so she is not going back to him.

During the rest of her pregnancy, Evita continues to "have fun," and has no more prenatal check-ups. She is an alcoholic. She is even quite drunk the night her labor pains start and she goes to the hospital. Her child is born with fetal alcohol syndrome. Although it has normal features (not all do), it has a heart murmur and could be retarded. The physicians notify the local Children's Aid Society which starts action to gain custody of the child. The Crown Attorney is considering prosecuting Evita for child abuse. Is she guilty?

18. Gwen and her husband, Hoyt, are both somewhat mentally retarded and have the emotional development of people thirteen years old. A year ago they received a check for $2,000 due to previous mistakes in

welfare payments. They immediately spent it all to make down payments on furniture and to buy an expensive cat. A month later the welfare workers found the cat dead of starvation. A couple of months after that, all their furniture was repossessed because they had not made any payments. Gwen has just given birth to a baby. Both Gwen and Hoyt are excited about the baby and are looking forward to taking it home. However, an agency has started proceedings to take the child from them. Is it unethical for Gwen and Hoyt to have children? Should the law remove the child from their custody? Why or why not?

19. Inez is twenty-five years old; her husband Jason is over fifty. Inez has just given birth to a baby girl. However, the baby is rushed to the intensive care nursery when she is seen to have many defects. One of the baby's defects prevents feeding unless it has surgery. The infant has trisomy 13, one of the most severe genetic disorders and is unlikely to live even with surgery. Inez confides to the physician that Jason is not the baby's natural father, and she refuses consent for surgery. Is it ethically wrong not to perform surgery on the infant? Should the natural (genetic) father have a say in the treatment decision?

20. Although Kay is married to Lester, she is not living with him. Three months ago she left Lester and their two children to move in with Marvin. Kay gives birth to an infant with spina bifida and hydrocephalus. The lesion is low in the back, and the baby has some feeling in its legs and appears to be of normal intelligence. Marvin is its genetic father. However, when Kay learns that Lester is legally responsible for the baby and must pay the medical bills, she refuses permission for the physician to operate on the baby. The physicians go to court to get a legal order giving them permission to operate. However, because Lester and Kay now live in different counties, it is unclear which court has jurisdiction. After two-and-a-half months the legal issues are settled and the doctors given permission to operate. However, during the delay the baby has deteriorated and is more paralyzed than it would have been had surgery been performed immediately. Moreover, it is now mildly retarded. Is it ethical for Kay to refuse to consent to surgery? Should Lester be legally responsible for the infant? Are the courts the appropriate organization to decide this case? If so, what, if anything, should be done to speed such a decision? If not, who should make the decision?

21. Noelle is born prematurely on December 27th. She weighs only 1435 grams (3 lbs. and 2½ oz.) and is about twenty-nine weeks gestation. To make matters worse, she has a heart defect that requires surgery. The doctor in charge brags to her parents, Orson and Phyllis, that he never gives up on babies. He always does everything in his power to bring them through. At first Orson and Phyllis are comforted by these comments. But as the days go by, the doctor's words come to haunt them. The surgery on the heart is successful, but Noelle develops an infection and respiratory distress. She is put on a ventilator and given antibiotics. Her heart stops twice, but she is resuscitated. She is declining very slowly. When further breathing complications develop, the doctors perform a tracheostomy. By this point Orson and Phyllis do not believe that she has a chance to live. They cautiously ask the doctor to stop heroic treatments. However, he says, "Don't you care for your baby? What kind of parents are you, anyway?" After two more weeks, Noelle finally dies. Orson and Phyllis are given a hospital bill for $34,559, of

which their insurance will pay $25,000. Should all of this treatment have been given to Noelle? If not, when should efforts to save her life have ceased? Who should decide when to stop? If the treatment should have been provided, who should pay the bill?

22. The doctors tell Rosa and Sidney that their new baby boy has problems. He has Down syndrome which will produce mental retardation, although they cannot be sure how bad. Such children, however, are trainable and, with proper care, happy and loving. He also has a heart condition which does not pose an immediate problem although it may cause problems later. The immediate problem is a blockage that prevents food from getting through the intestinal tract. The physicians request permission to operate. After anguished discussion, Rosa and Sidney decide not to give permission for the operation. However, the physicians apply to a court for permission to operate and it is given. Two weeks after the surgery, the infant is sent home with Rosa and Sidney. Is the decision by Rosa and Sidney unethical? Should the court have ordered the surgery? Is it ethical or proper for a court to order surgery and then return the infant to the care of Rosa and Sidney? If not, what should be done when courts order such treatment?

Scenarios

23. Tammy is dying of leukemia. She does not want to die; she is only twenty-three years old and has much to live for. She and Upton were planning to marry this summer. One day a doctor comes to her and says that he would like to try an experiment on her. If successful, she will live. He wants to take one of her eggs. He will treat it so that it will start reproducing. It will not really be a fertilized embryo, he insists, because it will not be fertilized. However, it will grow like one. If he can culture it to about twelve days, he will have the beginning cells for bone marrow. If he cultures these cells and then uses them to replace those in her bone marrow, there may be enough new cells to work properly and cure her leukemia. If Tammy consents, is this experiment ethical?

24. Victoria is in the hospital to have an abortion. She is fifteen weeks pregnant. A research scientist approaches her and asks whether he can have her fetus. He explains that he would like to have it whole, and that it would be better if she had a hysterotomy with general anesthesia. But if she is unwilling to undergo this operation, he would still like the fetus. He would like to try to see if he can bring the fetus to full development in the laboratory. If he is successful, he will put the infant up for adoption. She will have no responsibility for the infant. If the fetus lives but does not develop successfully, he will let it die. Would it be wrong for Victoria to consent? If she does, is the experiment ethically permissible?

Index

Note: Boldface page numbers indicate basic discussions of a topic as opposed to other references.